Runes: Healing and Diet

Sigrún Gregerson

Runic Consultant:
Freya Aswynn

Second printing

Cover image is from Freya Aswynn.

ISBN: 9798656849760

For those interested in Rune lessons with Freya Aswynn, you can get in contact with her via her email : faswynn@yahoo.com

Freya's Facebook page: https://www.facebook.com/FreyaAswynnOfficialFanpage/

Freya's website: http://aswynn.com/?fbclid=IwAR0C-zPgEq8P15hh0zf_Ms1N6ER5u-Rxo4Jx7LD3UXgk-_w6m3RVTc9GIBc

Sigrún Gregerson can be found online on Facebook: https://www.facebook.com/SigrunGregerson/

Sigrún's Instagram: https://www.instagram.com/sigrungregerson/

Dedicated to
my son, Bjorn Erik

A Blessing of Health

To the person reading this book: May your journey to a healthy body and an enlightened mind bring you to Wunjo. Your first Othala is your body, so may all of your exercises bring you Uruz and Sowilo. Lastly, may your study of the runic mysteries lead to Gebo of Kenaz and Ansuz.

Table of Contents

1. Introduction   Page 10

2. What are the Runes?   Page 18

3. Runes and Other Correspondences
Page 46

4. Runic Diet   Page 70
5. Herbs, Runes, and the Gods
Page 75
6. Runic Food, Vitamins and Minerals
Diet Friendly Recipes   Page 99

7. Diet Friendly Recipes   Page
110
8. Sigrun's Diet Diary   Page 121
9. Further Knowledge   Page 135

"Runes: Healing and Diet" is a wonderful integration of the sacred runes' strength and energy to help empower healing. The healing energy of the runes has not been explored deeply enough, but here in this book, they are. This book will unlock the keys to heal you- mind, body, and spirit and help guide you on your path to a healthier diet and achieve your desired weight loss goals. In this book, Sigrun has laid out an easy to follow and maintain diet and exercise plan. The meals suggested are perfectly balanced for those seeking to feel full but not break the diet. This book is an achievement in health, healing, and well-being. I will soon be using Tiawaz during sparing and Uruz for post workouts.

Hrafnar Gregerson - Master of Martial Arts: 4th degree Black Belt in Tae Kwon Do, 3rd Degree Black Belt Jiu-Jitsu, Competitive Dutch Thai Kick Boxing.

1. Introduction

I first discovered the magick of runes with Freya Aswynn's book "<u>Northern Mysteries and Magick</u>" in 2016. I had a grounding in the Norse tradition and myths already, but I never had a magick system that worked for me. The runes were the answer to this. After reading Freya's book, I was soon using rune magick in my daily life and with great success!

It was only when after I had my first baby that I had to use runes for healing along with medical care. With a new use of runes being discovered, I set out to learn more. I wanted to use runes in every area of my life. In 2019, I saw Freya promoting rune teaching on Facebook and for only $35! I couldn't pass this up! I took several weeks of classes before we came up with an idea for a book.

The contents of this book are a result of our discussions of the aspects of the runes to healing, health, food, and diet. The runes and the northern mysteries are well suited for health benefits, mental and physical. With these ideas, I also started a diet that would correspond with the runes and the Gods of the Norse pantheon.

Sigrún's Runic Healing Story

I had just given birth to my son, Bjorn, who was 9 pounds at birth. He was my first child and my pregnancy was normal and I had no complications other than having a large child due to my husbands' Frisian heritage. I had no gestational diabetes either.

Given Bjorn was larger in the womb than what was normal, I had expressed concern to the midwives that my child would be too large and I would have to have a c-section. I did not want one. I asked that they induce labor early, they declined, saying that they could not due to the hospital's policy. This was just another way to make the hospital look good by having low c-section rates.

I accepted this as a hard truth. When I went into labor, it lasted nearly 30 hours. I had an epidural, having every intention to deliver naturally, but due to Bjorn being a big baby, it wasn't possible without causing him physical damage. The doctor on call (I had not seen an actual MD in my entire pregnancy) told me this and that I would have to have a c-section. I was scared but went in for it anyway, as to not cause nerve damage to Bjorn or myself.

I remember being carted into the OR, visualizing the Berkana rune. In hindsight, I should have also focused on Algiz for protection. Because what happened a few days after the c-section was terrible. We found out that I had a small bowel obstruction. So I had to be transported to another hospital in town for the surgery (the hospital I was at only did L&D).

With the surgery being done, it looked like someone had tried to gut me, but then gave up. The surgeon said, "Oh, it's only a small incision" which left a nearly 4 inch Isa rune on me. But this surgery didn't fix the problem and I was stuck in the hospital for another 14 days.

I had an NG tube, a PICC line, a TPN, 2 different drains out of my gut because of an infection, multiple antibiotic treatments that didn't work (one I was allergic to and had to inform the MD's myself) and to top it all off, a blood clot, thanks to the PICC line! I was on my third antibiotic, 16 days into the ordeal, my husband was having to care for our newborn by himself (he was also a first-time father). I broke down, then focused my energy into the Uruz rune and played Wardruna's song

'UruR', which is the Uruz rune song. The next day, my white blood cell count was down, and I was discharged from the hospital.

*A Note on the spelling 'Magic' in this book. It is apart of my tradition and the tradition of many others to spell magic with a 'K'. This comes from Aleister Crowley, who wanted to differentiate ritual 'Magick' from performance 'Magic'.

A Note on the Coronavirus

As this book is being written, we are in the middle of a world wild pandemic. Covid 19, also known as the Coronavirus. It has gone from being a small news story in China in December 2019 to changing the world forever as of March 2020.

The threat of sickness and disruption has impacted everyone. We are all being encouraged or even forced to stay home. Local businesses and restaurants closed but will make delivery and no social gatherings over 50 people (here in Washington State). We have been recommended staying 6 feet away from other people. Grocery stores had panic rushes on them, some of them being out of toilet paper for several weeks. There are even shortages of medical supplies, people are being asked to make masks at home for medical staff and themselves.

The threat will not pass quickly. In terms of diet and exercise, keep at it. A healthy body will keep you alive if you get the virus. Keep food on hand that benefits the immune system, wash your hands but also moisturize. Overly dry hands can lead to other problems such as causing fissures in the skin that lead to infections. It is also advisable to keep your fingernails trimmed, bacteria can be underneath your nails, viruses too.

The cause of this virus is up for debate still. Hagalaz is playing a role for sure. Things will not change quickly. Keep your health in check, Uruz. Protect your family, Algiz. Preserve your voice and your lungs, Ansuz.

2. What Are The Runes?

While runes were originally used as a writing system, they were also used in magick of all sorts. runes have been used for healing in the past and weight loss draws from that. While the Scandinavians and Vikings didn't have a lot of weight problems (being fat was a luxury), in modern times we do.

Spirituality and religion evolves overtime, thus magick does as well. It is not too much of a stretch to take the runes to a new application, while keeping their traditional meanings intact.

How to use the runes in healing

A note before we get started: Do not use runes for healing as a substitute for medical care. Use them in conjunction with medical care that is being provided by a healthcare provider.

You can use runes for healing in a variety of different ways.

Visualization: Picture the rune in your mind or/and on your body. For example, if you are having back pain, visualize Uruz, and Eihwaz. Uruz taking away the pain, and Eihwaz straightening your back.

Chanting: Chanting the runes is an ancient art. It's called Galdr, and is an invocation of the runes power and a form of meditation as well. To do this, speak the name of the rune but vibrate your voice while you're doing it. Also, have the tone of your voice match the energy of the rune. For example, during my warfarin treatment, I would chant Raidho and Laguz. I would speak Raidho like "Raaaaaeeee-dooo" several time, then Laguz would sound out like "Laaaaaaaaaaaaaguuuuuuzzzzz."

Writing: You can write or draw a rune onto a piece of paper and carry it with you. An example is if you are starting a diet, you want to remind yourself of the transformation, draw Dagaz on a piece of paper and take it with you to work or where ever to remind yourself. You can also get creative with food in this way. You can draw an Ansuz rune over a cooking meal, using visualization, to bless the meal with that rune. You can also draw the rune on food with a knife, such as a piece of steak or potato, before you cook it to eat the rune to ingest its power.

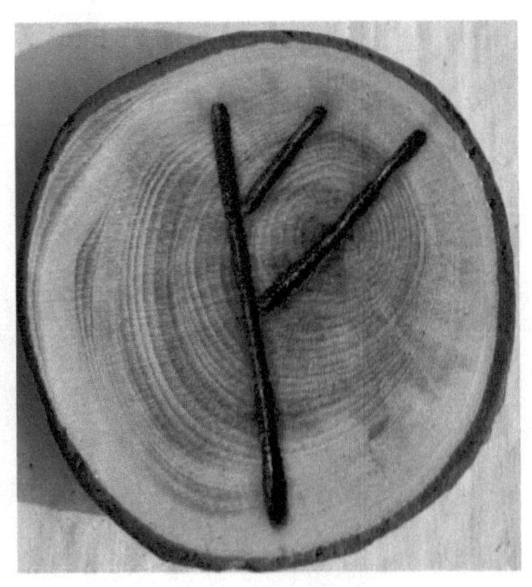

<u>Fehu</u>

The traditional meaning of this rune is wealth and cattle. Cattle have always been associated with wealth, even today having 40 head of cattle is equated to a pretty penny. Fehu is also associated with movable wealth, which is what cattle are.

Suggested application: Digestive healing, body improvement via proper diet and exercise. Weight gain after chemo/radiation or other cases of disease-related weight loss.

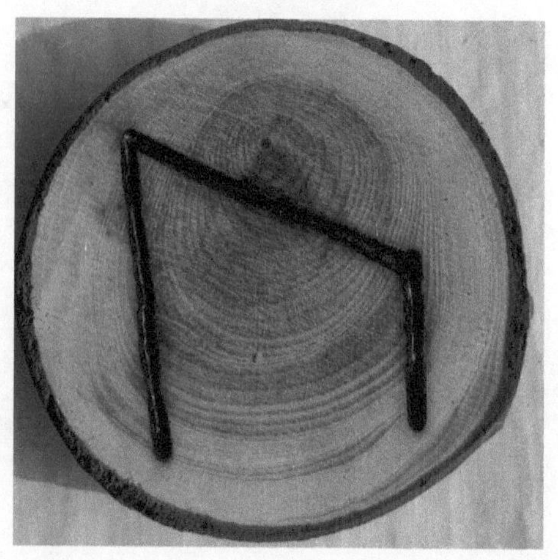

<u>Uruz</u>

Uruz is associated with health and primal strength of the ancient auroch. It is the go-to rune for healing and strength.

Suggested application: Treating infections, even sepsis! See Sigrun's story for more. Use Uruz to strengthen the body during and after an illness. Also, use Uruz to enhance the body as you are working out. Uruz can be used for those undergoing cancer treatment.

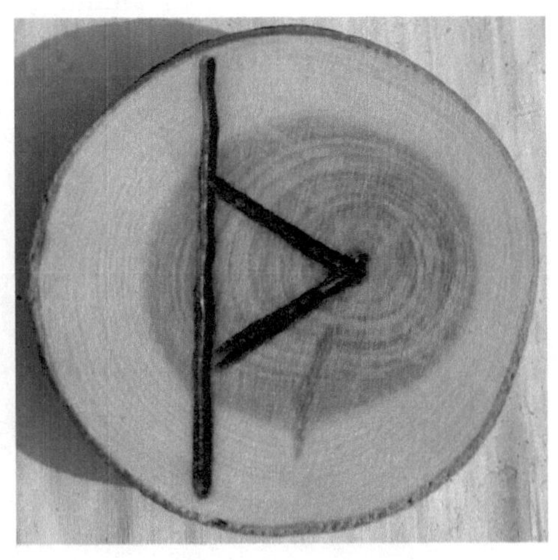

Thurisaz

This rune is associated with giants and Thor's hammer, Mjölnir. It is quite an aggressive rune but also has its protective qualities. It is associated with thorns, and what is the point of a thorn? To protect the plant from animals eating it.

Suggested application: Use for protection against an aggressive illness. Use this carefully.

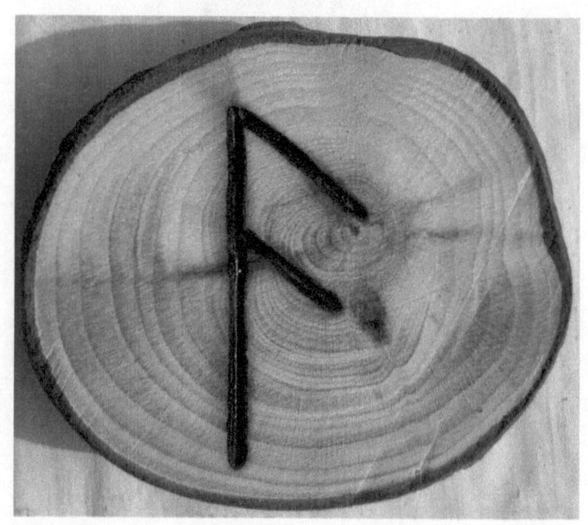

<u>Ansuz</u>

This rune is the rune of Odin. It is associated with communication and intelligence, thus your lungs, speech, throat, and your brain.

Suggested application: Helpful for asthma, throat issues, throat irritation, and mental health.

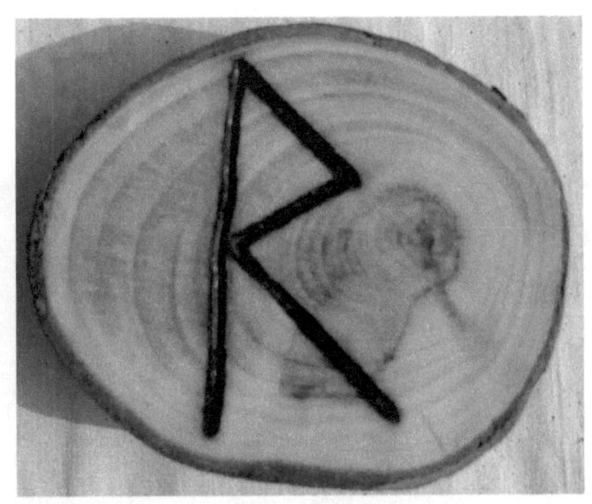

Raidho

The meaning of this rune is "riding," such as a journey. It also refers to anything that takes a path, such as food in your body or your blood.

Suggested application: Blood clots (under the direct care of blood thinners). I used this myself when I was on warfarin for five months. Raidho is also useful for digestive issues.

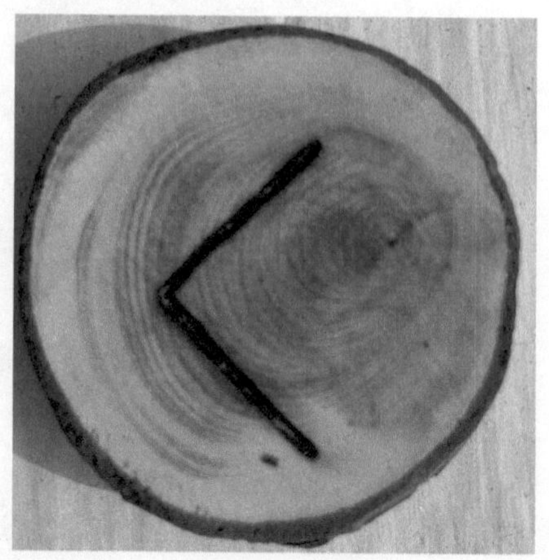

<u>Kenaz</u>

Kenaz is traditionally referred to as a torch or light. It is also associated with knowledge.

Suggested application: Kenaz can be used as a visualization over your healthcare providers along with Ansuz, so they focus and use their best knowledge.

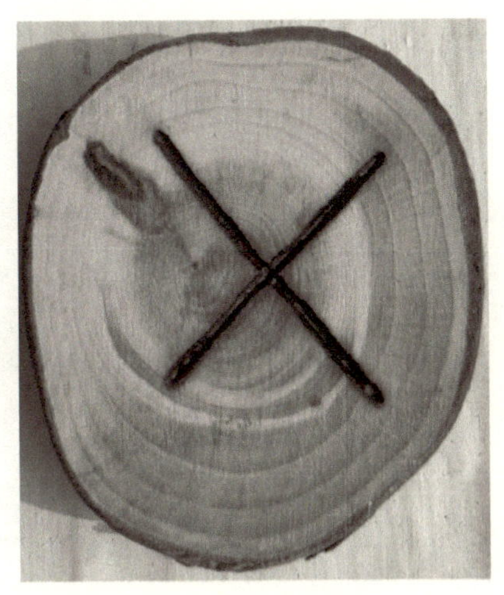

Gebo
Non-invertible Rune

Gebo, a wonderful rune. It's meaning is 'gift.' It also is associated with balance. It is a rune that cannot be inverted, but it can be negatively aspected.

Suggested application: Correct diet that is nourishing the body.

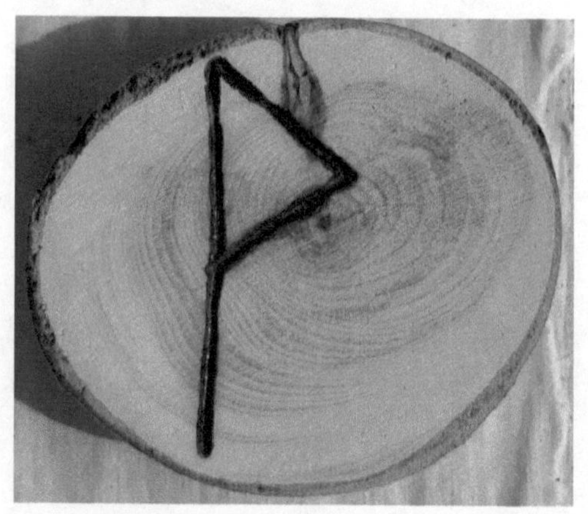

<u>Wunjo</u>

Wunjo's traditional meaning is 'Joy'; it can be associated with positive emotions and enjoyment.

Suggested application: It can help with emotional healing and nerve pain. It works well for sciatic nerve pain.

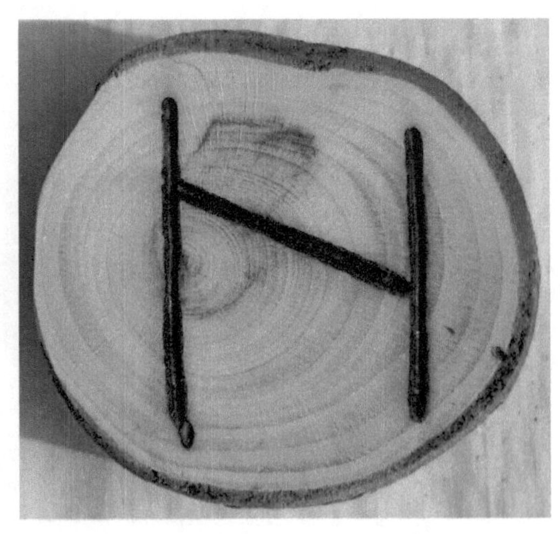

<u>Hagalaz</u>

The traditional meaning of this rune is 'Hail.' Anyone that has seen a hail storm can say it's destructive and frightening, but it can cause change.

Suggested application: It may point to mental diseases or diseases caused by addiction. For this, seek psychological healing.

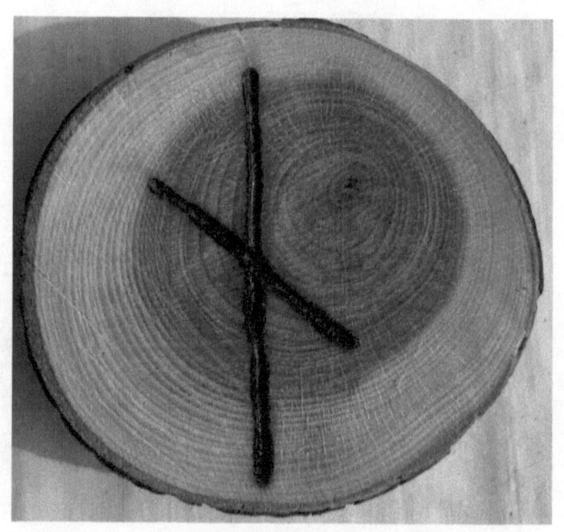

<u>Nauthiz</u>
<u>*Non-invertible rune*</u>

Nauthiz means "Need", as in what NEEDS to be done.

Suggested application: Advised to assess in what NEEDS to be done with your health.

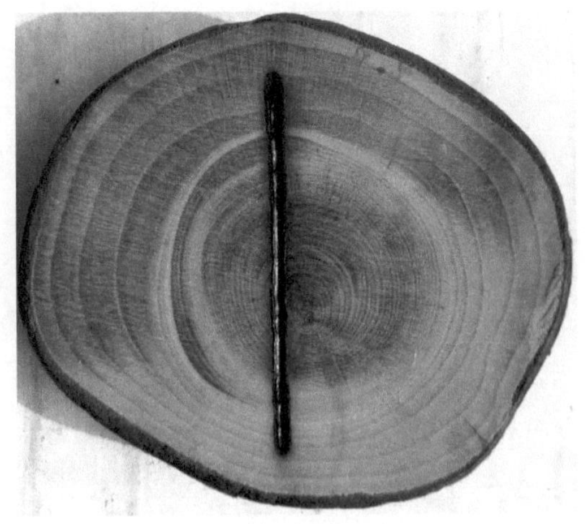

<u>Isa</u>
<u>*Non-invertible rune*</u>

Isa is a simple rune with a deep meaning. It's traditional meaning is "Ice". It is stagnation but also consistency, like ice glacier.

Suggested application: Halting high fever or aggressive cancers. It also works on a burn.

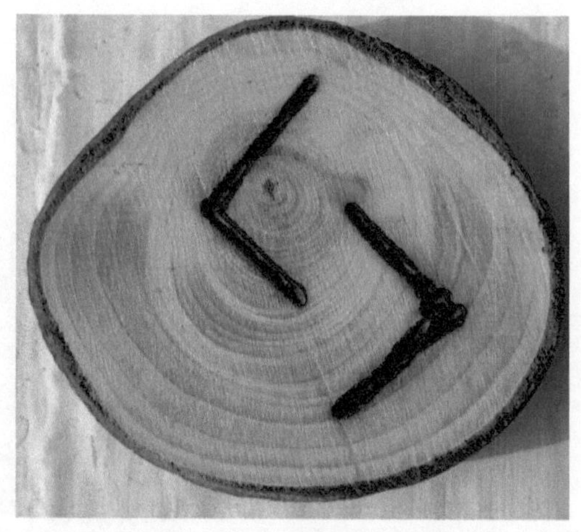

<u>Jera</u>
<u>Non-invertible rune</u>

Jera's traditional meaning is "Year" or "Harvest." Jera represents the passage of time, therefor digestion, which does take time.

Suggested application: Healthy gut bacteria. Also healing over time (pair with appropriate rune).

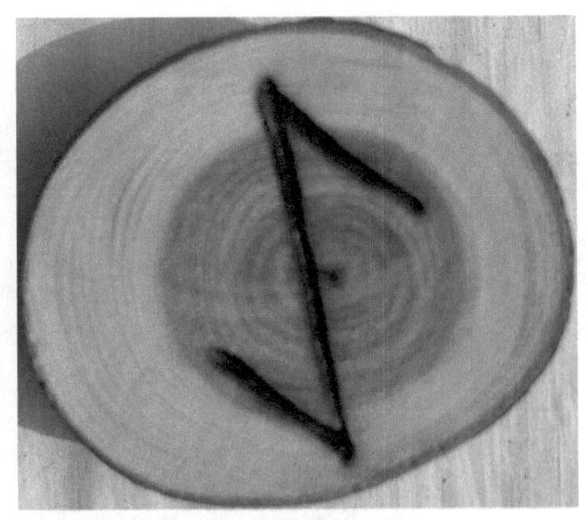

Eihwaz
Non-invertible rune

Eihwaz means "Tree" or "Yew" and is associated with Yggdrasil, the world tree of the Norse. Yggdrasil holds the nine worlds in its branches, just like your bones hold your body up and protects your vital organs.

Suggested application: It can be seen as a symbol of the spine and within the spine the central nervous system

This rune can help with back and skeletal strength.

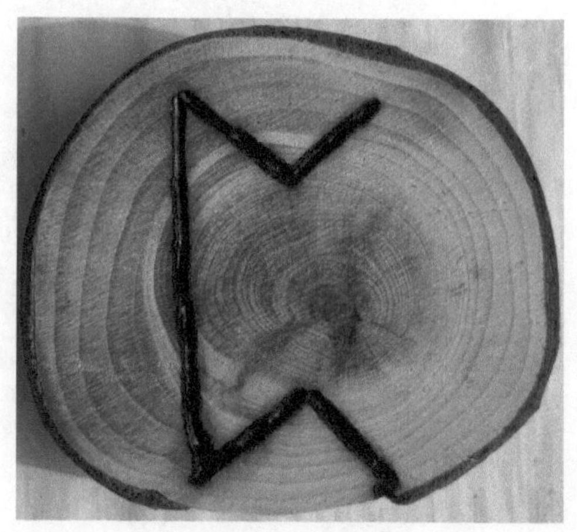

Perthro

Perthro symbolized anything unknown but also represents the womb or uterus.

Suggested application: Helpful for feminine health and a healthy menstrual cycle. Pair with Uruz, Berkana and Algiz for a safe birth.

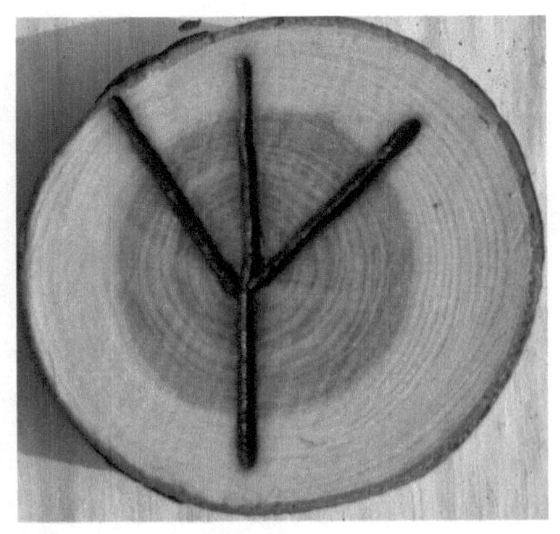

<u>Algiz</u>

Algiz's traditional meaning is "Protection," it is THE best rune for protection and it connects us to the Gods.

Suggested application: It can protect the whole body and all its systems. It also offers protection against disease, as well as protection against medical malpractice. Pair with appropriate rune if for example, when going in for surgery.

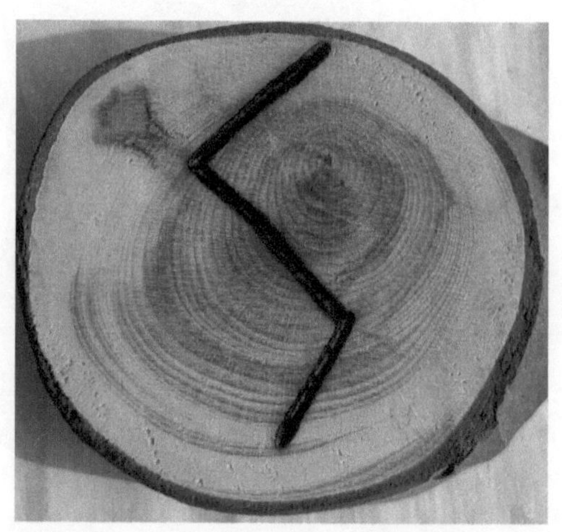

Sowulo
Non-invertible rune

Sowulo's traditional meaning is "Sun," and the sun gives us energy, even the energy to accomplish what you need to do. This rune is also associated with victory.

Suggested application: This rune is also associated with Health is general, life force and Vitamin D3.

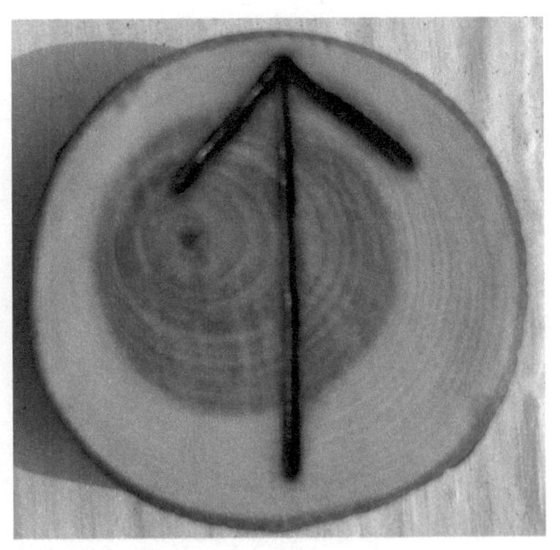

Teiwaz

Teiwaz is named after the God Tyr, the god of Justice. This rune is associated with warriors and law and is also associated with men, as it is shaped like a phallus. It is also associated by correspondences to the T cells of the immune system.

Suggested application: Fighting cancer, any therapy that involves male fertility issues, and injectable medications of any kind. It also strengthening ones immune system.

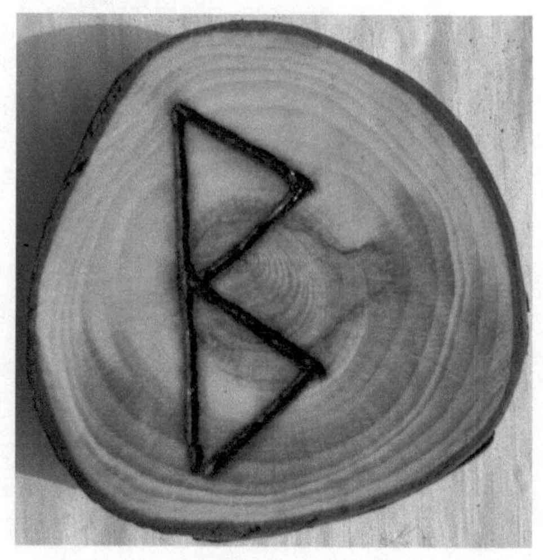

<u>Berkana</u>

Berkana's traditional meaning is "Birch" as in the birch tree. This rune is also associated with Goddesses, women, children, and childbirth.

Suggested application: Female fertility and breast health.

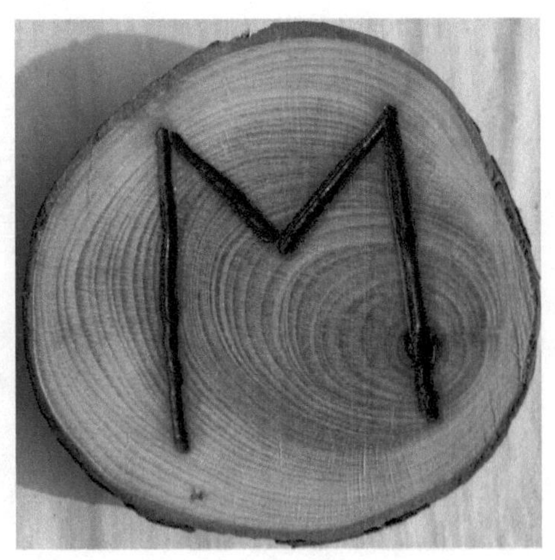

Ehwaz

This runes traditional meaning is "Horse." While most people don't have a horse, this rune has to do with transportation that a horse would provide, like a car or a bus.

Suggested application: Healthy movement of bowels and muscles.

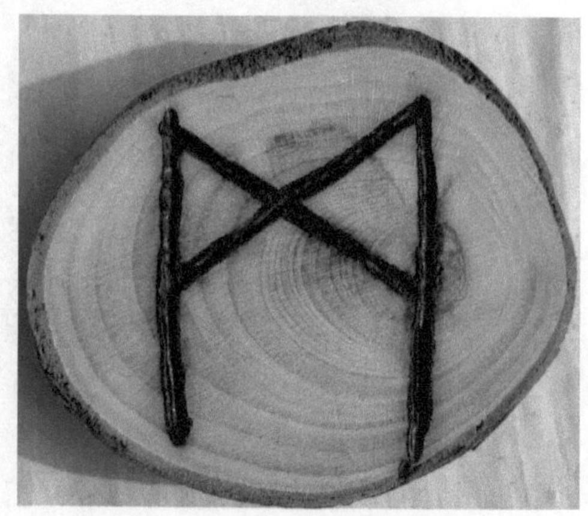

<u>Mannaz</u>
This runes traditional meaning is "Man." It is associated with the mind.

Suggested application: Mental relationship changes or treatment (improving relationships). Also, Parkinson's disease, treating nerve damage (pair with Ansuz or Ehwaz)

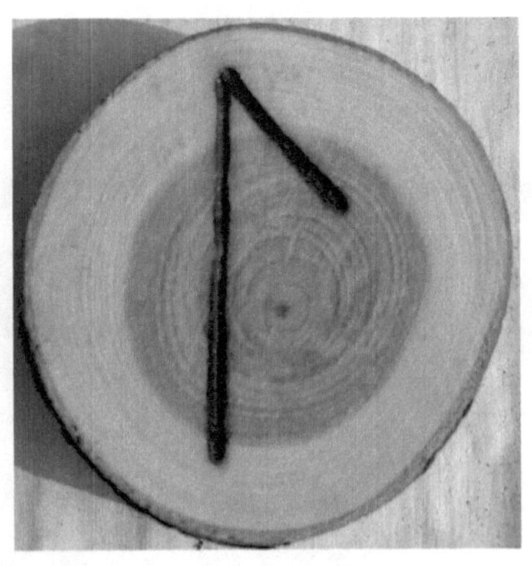

Laguz

The traditional meaning of Laguz is "Lake" or "Water." A primary health fact is that water is good for you, but water is also associated with emotions, as is this rune.

Suggested application: Emotional issues and resolving blood clots in addition to medication. I have used this during my warfarin therapy.

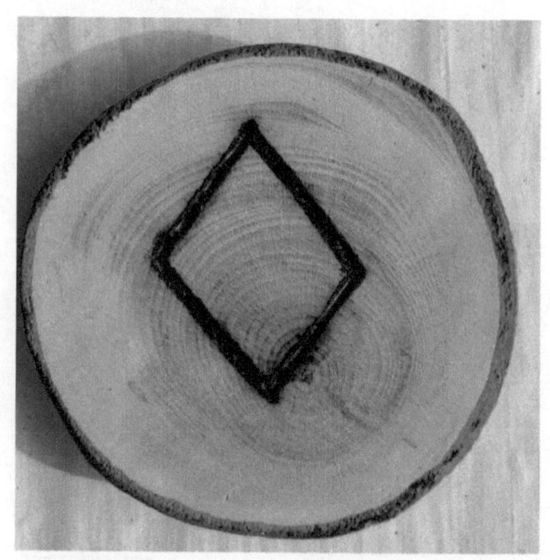

Inguz
Non-invertible Rune

This rune is associated with male fertility and agriculture. It is also associated with the God Freyr.

Suggested application: Potent male fertility, fertility treatment for males and prostate health

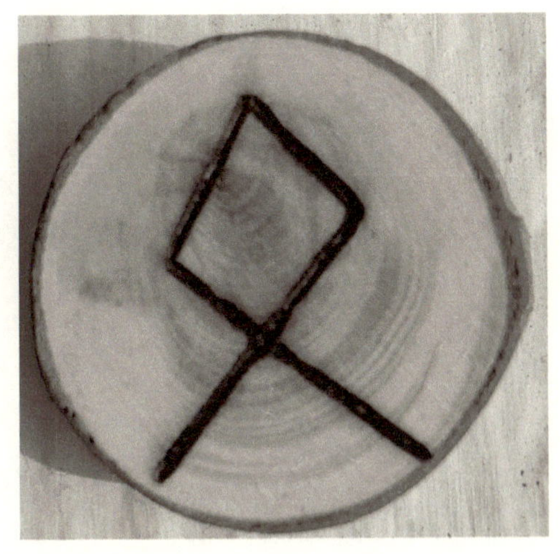

<u>Othala</u>

Othala's traditional meaning is "Inherited land." It is also associated with one's family and ancestors. So it can be related to health-wise with any illnesses that run in the family.

Suggested application: Family diseases, such as cancers that run in the family. Also, positive family health attributes.

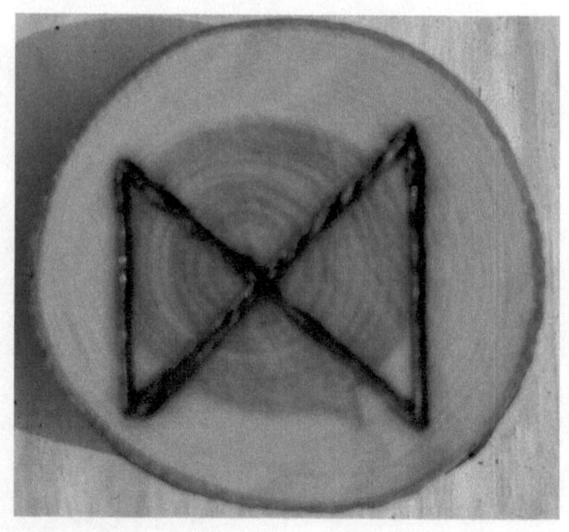

<u>Dagaz</u>
<u>Non-invertable Rune</u>

The traditional meaning of this rune is "Day." It's associated with changes and transformation.

Suggested application: Psychical transformation from a healthy diet.

Useful for: Diet change, lifestyle change.

3. Runic and Other Correspondences

The following pages are a culmination of runic correspondences of health, herbs, and the Norse Gods. With a basic understanding of the runes, we can pinpoint a lack of or overabundance of a specific rune in relation to health.

It is important to note that runic healing should only be used in combination with professional medical care and advice. Get a diagnosis first. Do not substitute the information in this book for professional medical care from your healthcare provider.

Nine Systems of the body to the Nine Worlds

In this book, many references and correspondences will be made not only to the runes but to the Nine Worlds in the Norse Cosmos. If the reader of this book in unfamiliar with the Nine Worlds, this section will serve as a very brief explanation.

Midgard: The realm of humanity, our own home.

Asgard: The realm of the Aesir, the war tribe of Gods. In this realm is where many halls of the Gods are located, including the famous Valhalla. This is also the realm that is associated with Odin and higher planes of consciousness.

Vanaheim: The realm of the Vanir gods, the fertility Gods of the Norse. This realm is also associated with magick and animals.

Alfaheim: This is the realm of light elves and is ruled by one of the Vanir, Freyr.

Jotunheim: The realm of the Jotun, the giants. This is a realm of chaos and magick.

Swartalfheim: The realm of the dark elves or dwarves. This realm is below Midgard.

Niflheim: This is the realm of ice that existed at the time of creation of the cosmos.

Muspelheim: The realm of fire and ruled by the giant Surt, the greatest enemy of the Aesir.

Helheim: This is the land of the dead, but it is not like the Christian 'Hell' in any way. Helheim is incredibly cold, and those who die from natural causes, sickness, or old age go here, but it is not a punishment. The Goddess Hel rules it.

Now we can compare the 9 worlds to the 9 systems of the body.

Skeletal System: Midgard is the world we live on, the realm of humanity, our home, our Othala. Your bones are your home, your Othala! Your ribs protect your vital organs, and your home protects you from the elements.

Digestive System: We can connect to Swartalfheim is the world of the dwarves or dark elves. Your digestive system processes your food into energy, much as the dwarves create beautiful things out of ore and gems. Swartalfheim is also the realm of transformation.

Lymphatic System: Can be associated with Asgard, the world of the Aesir Gods. The Gods protect the nine worlds (each in their own way or for their own interest). The lymphatic system protects the body from infection.

Muscle System: We connected to Jotunheim, the world of the Jotun, also known as the giants. Giants are known for their strength. Your muscles carry your body and are your strength.

Respiratory System: Can be associated with Alfheim, known for its forests. On earth, our forests create the oxygen that we breathe. They are the lungs of the planet. Thus Alfheim can be connected to the respiratory (lungs) system.

Endocrine System: Niflheim is the world of ice but also water.
When Niflheim and Muspeleim converged in the Ginnungagap, the void, and the heat of Muspeleim melted Niflheims ice. Then from the ice, Ymir, the first Jotun, emerged, and so did the cow, Audumla. Through these entities, the creation of the other worlds and life happened. Thus with the Endocrine system creates growth and produces hormones. It has the potential to create and does so.

Nervous System: Helheim, the world of the dead, because even for a little bit after death, our nerves are still firing. Our nervous system also alerts us to spirits around us, so we connect it to the nervous system.

Circulatory System: We can connect to Muspeleim, which is the world of fire. Its part in the creation of the Norse cosmos is essential because it's fires melted the ice of Niflheim. The circulatory system and the Endocrine system work together as well. The endocrine system creates hormones, and the Circulatory system transports them; the ice of Niflheim held Audumla and Ymir, the fires of Muspelheim released them.

Reproductive System: Vanaheim- The Vanir are Gods of nature and fertility, thus an easy link to the Reproductive system.

Chakras to the 9 Worlds

There are many people who are familiar with Chakras and healing. This section will help those people make associations with these energy centers and the runes.

We can look at the 9 non-investable runes and match them with the charkas as well. As an exercise, I recommend meditating on the runes and the chakras, because each rune resonates with a persons chakras on an individual level.

We can look at the nine non-invertible runes and match them with the chakras. As an exercise, I recommend meditating on the runes and the chakras because each rune resonates with a person's chakras on an individual level. They may even fluctuate from day-to-day!

For example, here is how I view my chakras to the nine non-invertible runes.

- For the energy center at the feet, I associate it with Isa.
- For my Root Chakra, Dagaz, as that rune symbolizes the hips and helps me feel balanced.
- The Sacral Chakra, Inguz. Because Inguz is associated with fertility and the sacral chakra is associated with female fertility (where the womb is).
- The Solar Plexus, Nauthiz, because I am most often in need of personal power.
- For the Heart Chakra, Gebo. Gebo means gift, and the heart guides most gifts I buy. I also associate Gebo with compassion.
- The Throat Chakra I associate with Hagalaz. It is an odd choice to some, but I regret somethings that I say, and Hagalaz is connected to the past.

- The Third Eye is Jera for me. Jera can be seen as a turning wheel of time.
- The Crown Chakra is Sowulo. Sowulo is the sun and is a source of energy, physically and spiritually.
- For the Chakra above the Crown, the Soul star some call it, I connect to Eihwaz. Eihwaz, I see as a ladder that I can use to search and explore other realms in meditation. Eihwaz is connected to Yggdrasil as well.

You can also associate the chakras with the nine worlds. Each person will have different answers. Freya and I both had different answers! Make it another exercise for your mind.

For example,

- At the Base/feet - Nifleheim
- Root Chakra - Helheim: This chakra connects to your security, basic needs, grounding. Midgard can also be associated here.

- Sacral Chakra- Vanaheim or Swartalheim: Relationships and sexuality.
- Solar Plexus Chakra- Swartalfheim, Jotunheim or Midgard: Emotion - vitality and taking control
- Heart Chakra- Midgard, our home, our Othila. This is the realm where we live and love.
- Throat Chakra- Asgard, closely linked to the rune Ansuz, which is associated with Odin and speech.
- Third Eye Chakra- Helheim/ Vanaheim/Alfheim - Imagination, visualization, and intuition.
- Crown Chakra - Asgard/Alfheim - awareness of higher consciousness and wisdom.
- Soul Star Chakra - Asgard or Muspelheim. Muspelheim being at the top and Niflheim being at the bottom, which come together in Ginnungagap. The soul star chakra is where spiritual energy enters the body, so an association can be made to Asgard.

The Brain

Mind over matter! Within our minds, we have the power to utilize the runes to better our lives. Below is correspondence for the areas of the brain and the runes.

The Right Hemisphere: Art, creativity, intuition, left-hand control. It can be connected to Odin's raven Munin, which means memory.
Runes associated with this hemisphere: Perthro and Algiz.
The Left Hemisphere: Analytic thought, logic, reasoning, and right-hand control- It can be associated with Odin's other raven Hugin, which means thought.
Runes associated with this hemisphere: Ansuz, Mannaz, and Jera

Dagaz connects the left and right hemispheres of the brain. The corpus callosum, which joins the left and right hemispheres can be compared the

Bifrost bridge, bridging the hemispheres together - This superb esoteric insight is from Freya.

For the rest of the Futhark, we will look at the lobes of the brain:

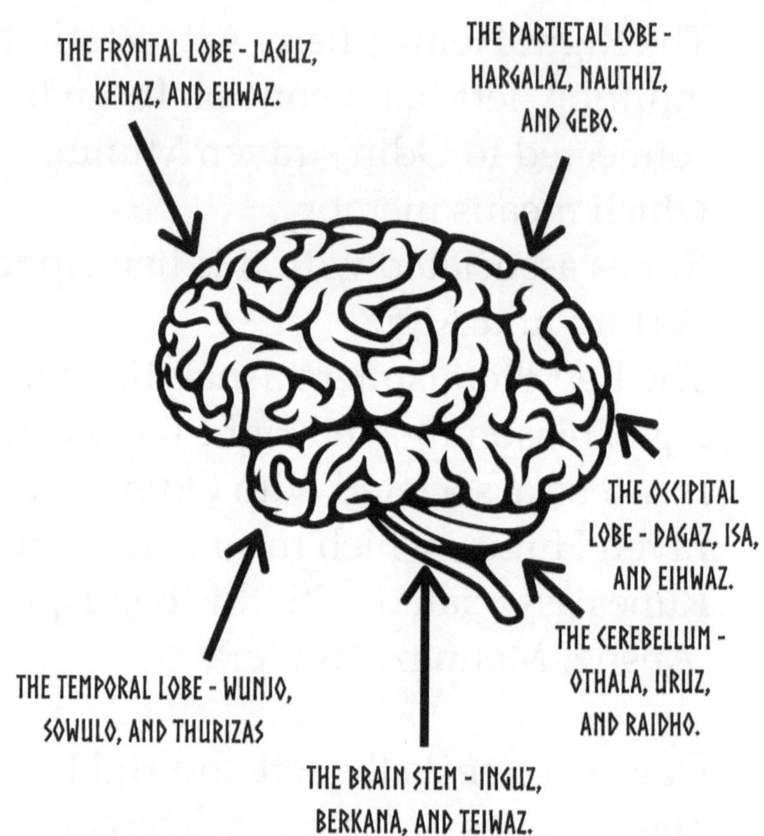

The Frontal Lobe - Problem-solving, emotional, reasoning, speaking, and voluntary motor activity.
Runic association: Laguz, Kenaz, and Ehwaz.

The Temporal Lobe - Understanding language, behavior, memory, and hearing.
Runic association: Wunjo, Sowulo, and Thurizas.

The Brain Stem: Breathing, alertness, sleep, and body functions
Runic association: Inguz, Berkana, and Teiwaz.

The Cerebellum: Balance, coordination, and muscle control.
Runic association: Othala, Uruz, and Raidho.

The Occipital Lobe: Vision and color vision
Runic association: Dagaz, Isa, and Eihwaz.

The Partietal lobe: Sensation, sensory perception, and reading.
Runic association: Hargalaz, Nauthiz, and Gebo.

A quick note on fight or flight responses for runic connections:
Fight - Teiwaz - The warrior rune
Flight - Berkana - The motherhood rune

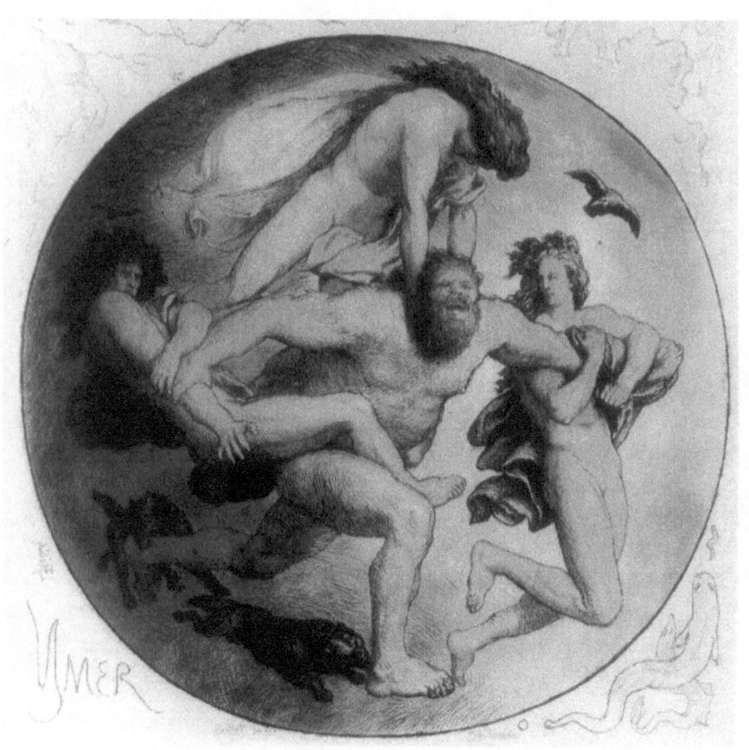

Of Bones and Runes
The First Giant Ymir, His Bones, and Our Bones

Ymir, the first giant, who was killed by Odin and his brothers. From Ymir's body, Odin and his brothers used his flesh to create the earth, from his sweat (or blood) the sea. From Ymir's bones, they created the mountains and used his hair to make the trees. To top it all off, Ymir's skull was fashioned into the sky.

Now in Ymir's dead flesh, there were maggots, and the 3 brothers took these maggots and made them into the Dwarves. Odin had 4 of the dwarves hold up the corners of Ymir's skull. So we have Nordri (North), Sundri (South), Austri (East) and Vestir (West).

Our own bodies are our world, your body is a temple, as they say. Your flesh is the earth, our Othala. Your blood and sweat is your sea, your Laguz. Your bones are your mountains, Eihwaz! Your hair is your trees and your skull is the sky, held up by 4 dwarves, your arms, and your legs.
Flesh - Earth Othala.
Sweat/blood- Sea, blood was already attributed to Laguz.
Mountains - Bone - bones/skeletal system attributed to Eihwaz.
Trees - hair - Fehu.

Skull- Sky, the 4 dwarves that hold his skull up Perthro and Gebo.

Now the four dwarves are Nordri, Sundri, Austri, Vestir. Their names translate to Northern, Southern, Eastern, and Western. In our own body, we can see the directions on the compass: our arms and legs. Our body is also the pentacle, with our head as the top of the star and our outstretched arms being the other four points.

The Spine to Runes

Your spine is separated into 3 parts, your lumbar, thoracic, and cervical. Your lumbar is your lower spine, L5 to L1. The thoracic spine is in the middle, where all your vital organs are, Th 12 to 1. Then your cervical spine is the top portion of your spine, C7 to C1, leading up to your skull.

A meditation can be done by focusing on your spine, starting at the base of your spine chanting Fehu slowly, then slowly moving through the Futhark, one by one, focusing on each corresponding part of the spine.

The meditation is beneficial for many things, back healing after surgery, mental and physical alignment, and mental clarity.

Since there are three parts of the spine, we can associate them with the Norns, Urd, Verdandi and Skuld.

Lumbar - Urd - "the past" root and second chakra - well of origin
Thoracic - Verdandi "what is presently coming into begin", the middle where all our organs are.
Cervical- Skuld "What shall be", the closest to your head, your brain which creates your future.

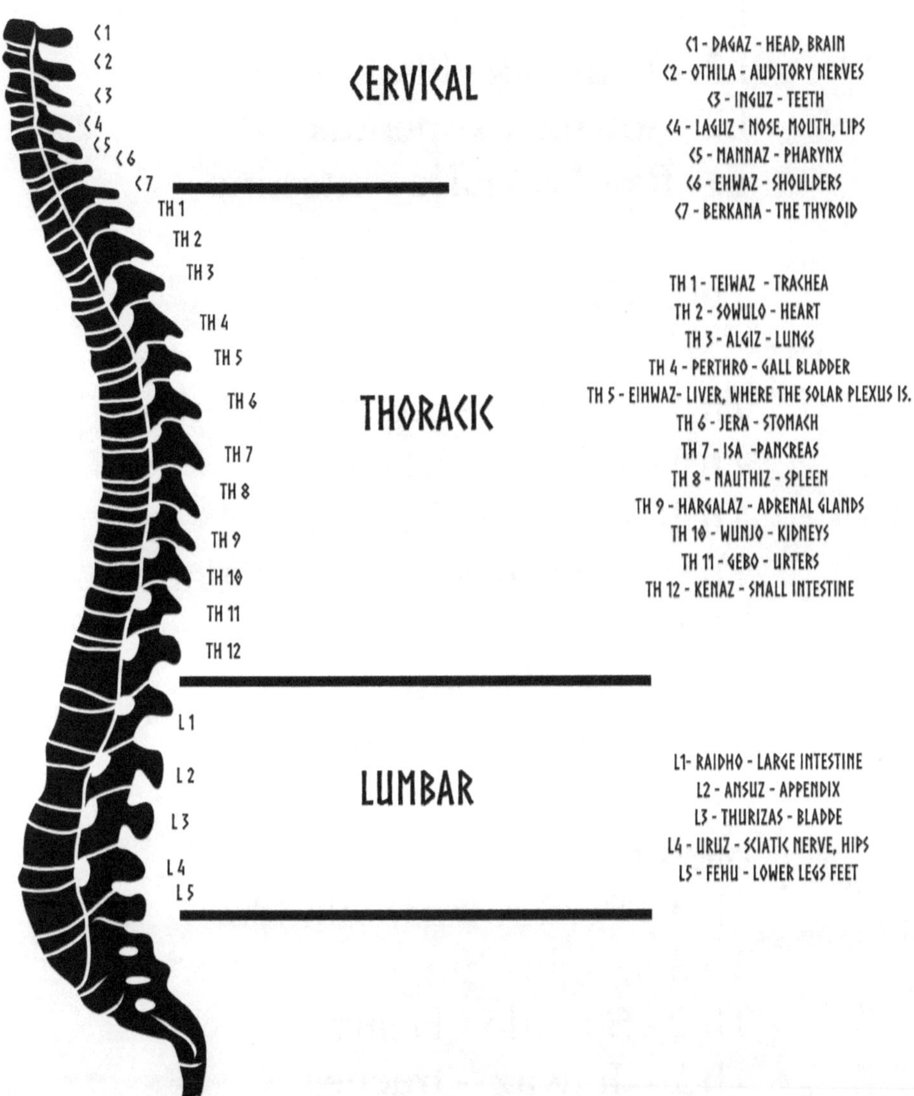
ᚲ1
ᚲ2
ᚲ3
ᚲ4
ᚲ5 ᚲ6
ᚲ7
TH 1
TH 2
TH 3
TH 4
TH 5
TH 6
TH 7
TH 8
TH 9
TH 10
TH 11
TH 12
L 1
L 2
L 3
L 4
L 5
CERVICAL
THORACIC
LUMBAR
ᚲ1 - DAGAZ - HEAD, BRAIN
ᚲ2 - OTHILA - AUDITORY NERVES
ᚲ3 - INGUZ - TEETH
ᚲ4 - LAGUZ - NOSE, MOUTH, LIPS
ᚲ5 - MANNAZ - PHARYNX
ᚲ6 - EHWAZ - SHOULDERS
ᚲ7 - BERKANA - THE THYROID
TH 1 - TEIWAZ - TRACHEA
TH 2 - SOWULO - HEART
TH 3 - ALGIZ - LUNGS
TH 4 - PERTHRO - GALL BLADDER
TH 5 - EIHWAZ- LIVER, WHERE THE SOLAR PLEXUS IS.
TH 6 - JERA - STOMACH
TH 7 - ISA - PANCREAS
TH 8 - NAUTHIZ - SPLEEN
TH 9 - HARGALAZ - ADRENAL GLANDS
TH 10 - WUNJO - KIDNEYS
TH 11 - GEBO - URTERS
TH 12 - KENAZ - SMALL INTESTINE
L1- RAIDHO - LARGE INTESTINE
L2 - ANSUZ - APPENDIX
L3 - THURIZAS - BLADDE
L4 - URUZ - SCIATIC NERVE, HIPS
L5 - FEHU - LOWER LEGS FEET

Lumbar

L5 - Fehu - Lower legs feet

L4 - Uruz - Sciatic nerve, hips

L3 - Thurizas - Bladder

L2 - Ansuz - Appendix

L1- Raidho - Large intestine

Thoracic spine

Th 12 - Kenaz - Small intestine

Th 11 - Gebo - Urters

Th 10 - Wunjo - Kidneys

Th 9 - Hargalaz - Adrenal glands

Th 8 - Nauthiz - Spleen

Th 7 - Isa -Pancreas

Th 6 - Jera - Stomach

Th 5 - Eihwaz- liver, where the solar plexus is.

Th 4 - Perthro - gall bladder

Th 3 - Algiz - lungs

Th 2 - Sowulo - Heart

Th 1 - Teiwaz - trachea

Cervical spine

C7 - Berkana - the thyroid
C6 - Ehwaz - Shoulders
C5 - Mannaz - Pharynx
C4 - Laguz - Nose, mouth, lips
C3 - Inguz - Teeth
C2 - Othila - Auditory nerves
C1 - Dagaz - Head, brain

4. Runic Diet

This next section will detail the out line of the diet for those who want to try it. You can try it for weight loss or health.

 The diet plan is half spiritual and half physical. You will be doing both meditations on the runes and diet/ exercise, and this diet is not a detox diet but focuses on calorie reduction. The calories you will eat will make you full and satisfied.

Diet Guidelines

Like any diet, this one has guidelines, though they are not extreme. Focus on keeping your carbohydrates low. This diet is not about carb counting, and it's not a Keto diet. You will need to limit eating bread, pasta, and sweets. Also, avoid heavy sugar drinks such as juice, sodas, beer, and wine. Make sure also to avoid processed cheap foods, as this is probably the reason you're reading this, and it's why I'm doing the diet as well.

With keeping carbs low, keep in mind how you feel, the first few days may be rough. If you feel overly hungry, listen to what your body wants, but if what your body wants is unhealthy, try to limit it.

What you will want to have a lot of in the diet is protein and animal fat. These will keep you level headed and satisfied. Beef, pork, chicken, venison, chicken, fish, and lamb. These are also nutrient-dense.

For a quick snack, cheese will be your best friend on this diet. Cheese from grass-fed cows is best, but if it's not available, conventional is fine. Goats cheese is excellent, too, if you like it. If you're lactose intolerant, peanut butter or cold cuts of meat will work. Eggs are also perfect for a quick snack if they are hard-boiled since they can be made ahead of time.

For those on a vegetarian diet, you may substitute as needed for meats. I must suggest you stay 'lacto vegetarian' and keep dairy in your diet, though, as you are cutting carbs, and you will need the animal fat to sustain yourself.

As for vegetables, carrots, celery, tomatoes, cauliflower, green beans, and anything else you like can be added to the diet, make sure you're not loading them up with ranch dressing or the like. A note on potatoes, they are acceptable but in moderation. At most, twice a week. Fruits are something else, though. Don't eat too many, as they are full of sugar, but an orange, banana, or avocado are suitable.

This diet does not involve any fasting. I knew from trying fasting diets before that it was impossible for me; I felt faint within 4 hours on those types of diets. When creating this diet, I understood that I could not be alone on this and that it could not a fasting diet.

Does this diet allow caffeine? Yes! One to two cups of coffee with real dairy creamer - no artificial creamer. Tea is also allowed.

Exercise

You cannot have a working diet without exercise. Luckily, it can be tailored to your capability. It can be anything on this diet as long as you are doing it. I mostly did walking with some weight resistance, using my own body by doing knee lifts. I also have a two-year-old who weighs 50 pounds, taking care of him is a work out of its own. So if you don't have kids, offer to babysit, you'll burn calories.

Another option is choosing a good work out program on YouTube. There are many to choose from. Pick anything that has spirts or bursts of effort, because this type of exercise will give you results quickly.

I also recommend having a pedometer to track your progress during workouts or walks. Most cell phones have a pedometer app for free or one built-in.

With your workouts, focus on your problem areas. For most people trying to lose weight, it might be their guts, and for others, it might be their arms or legs. For myself, I had to focus on my stomach, so knee lifts for me.

Example of exercises
Three sets of 10 knee lifts
1-mile walk
Three sets of 10 push-ups
Advance to more as you improve.

<u>5. Herbs, Runes, and the Gods</u>

Since the runes and the Gods of the Norse pantheon are so interconnected, it is essential to connect the two for guidance and inspiration for the diet. It may seem like a silly concept to some, but in the following pages, it will make more sense. For example, on Sundays, eat more vitamin C rich foods, and on Thursday, you will have a cheat day.

As it will be explained in the following pages, each day of the week corresponds with a Norse God or Goddesses. Six out of the seven days of the week are named after the Norse Gods, except for Saturday, which is named after Saturn.

Included in each day is a brief description of each God to acquaint those who are unfamiliar with them. There is also a poem to invoke the power of the God and a rune for a specific purpose. Poetry and Norse Gods go hand in hand!

For those of you who worship the Gods, you also may want to incorporate your better diet into the mix! Just sticking to a diet alone can be an offering to Gods. It shows commitment, improvement of yourself, and your wyrd. Our Gods want us to be the best versions of ourselves that we can be.

Sunday

Goddess association: Sunna or Sol
Goddess of the Sun, Sunna, or Sol, pulls the sun with her chariot and is chased by the wolves Skoll and Hati. These wolves will catch her during Ragnarok, destroying the sun.

- Herbal associations: Chamomile
- What to eat? Spicy foods, citrus fruits, and sunflower seeds as a treat.

"Sol, and swift and early riser!/The Sun herself
Sowulo and Raidho, help me to greet the day
Sol, driving swift and early riser!/Fast traveler
I lack in motivation
Show me how to move like I've got a hungry wolf behind me."

Monday

God association: Mani

Mani is the God of the Moon and the brother of Sol. He also drives a chariot while carrying the moon, which is chased by the wolves Skoll and Hati. His fate will be the same as his sister at Ragnarok.

- What to do and eat? On this day, start by looking up the phase the moon is currently occupying. If the moon is waxing, you can have an extra snack a day (following the diet guidelines). When the moon is waning, you will want to try to fast a little (what you can manage). The moon has its cycles, it waxes and wanes and our bodies wax and wane with our hormonal level changes (for both men and women).

Tuesday
God association: Tyr

God of justice, law, and war, his rune is Teiwaz which is associated with justice. Tuesday owes its name to this God.

Tyr is known for his role in the binding of the wolf Fenrir. This wolf was the son of Loki, and he grew so big the Gods became fearful of him, and only Tyr was brave enough to feed him. The Gods concluded that Fenrir needed to be tied down. They tried several different chains, each one failed, so they went to the dwarves for a solution. The dwarves of Svartalfheim created a ribbon made from things that cannot exist, or that you cannot see, such as the breath of a fish or a cat's footfalls. The Gods brought this ribbon to Fenrir, which the wolf thought of as pathetic. A ribbon cannot restrain a great wolf! Fenrir told the Gods that he would only allow them to bound him with the ribbon if one of them would stick their hand in his mouth, as a pledge of goodwill. The Gods knew the ribbon would indeed hold the wolf, so they were afraid to lose their hand, but Tyr came forward and placed his hand in Fenrir's open mouth. The Gods tied Fenrir with the ribbon, and the wolf tried to free himself. Only the harder he struggled, the tighter it got. Fenrir knew he had been tricked and bit off Tyr's hand.

- Herbal associations: Yarrow, Comfrey, Leek, and Onion (for wounded warriors)
- What to eat? Leek, onion, or fish for one meal in your day.
- What to do? This will be the day you will weigh yourself. Because of Tyr is the God of Justice, it's the correct time to put yourself on the scale.

Poem:
"This I will do/Teiwaz to make me strong
Fat I have become
This I will change/Tyr to keep me on the
path
I will change my ways in coming days
I will lose my extra pounds as a pledge
Gebo, the gift of health to myself"

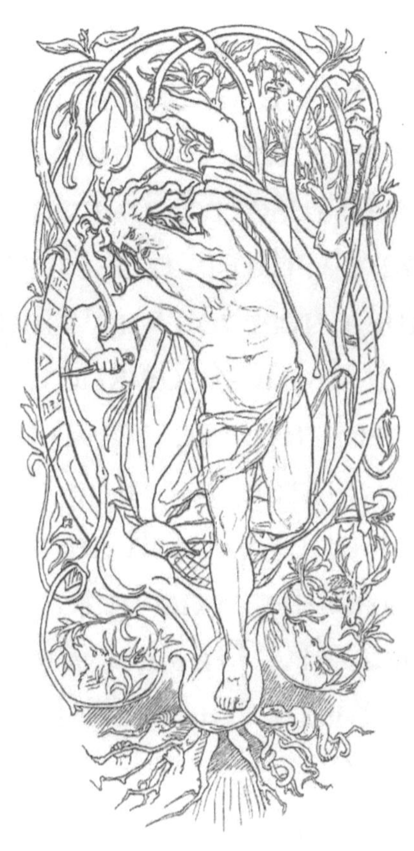

Wednesday
God association: Odin

Odin, leader of the Aesir, God of wisdom, war, and death. His rune is Ansuz.

Odin, known by many names, the All-Father, Hanged-God, One-Eyed, and many more. He is the second most recognizable Gods of the Norse

Pantheon behind his son Thor. Odin is a God of war but also of wisdom and death. There are many tales of Odin for you to research in your own time, but where Odin is most influential in my life is his quest for knowledge. In this never-ending quest for knowledge, Odin hung himself upside down on Yggdrasil, the worlds tree, for nine days, and acquired the Runes, which he then taught to Heimdallr, who in turn taught them to humanity. This act was of self-sacrifice. What will you sacrifice to attain your goals?

- Herbal associations: Pine, rosemary, eyebright
- What to eat? Beef or a vegetarian high protein. Walnuts as well (Walnut looks like the brain).
- What to do? Study diet and natural healing.

Poem:
"Odin's wisdom/ searching to expand
Ansuz concealed with fog
Odin's wisdom/ simple but wise
Bless this animal flesh (or non animal
protein.)
Eating well does the Ansuz well"

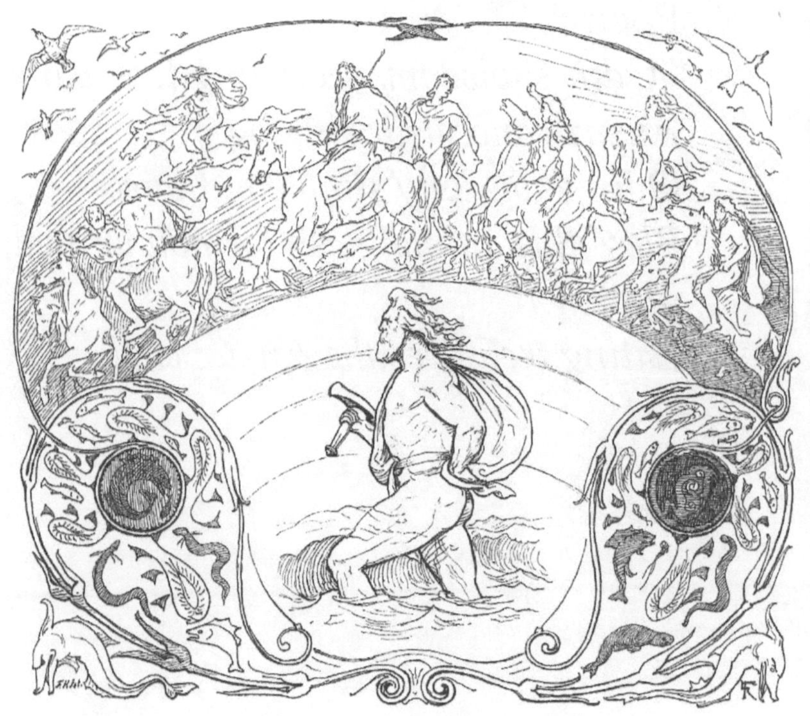

Thursday

God association: Thor

This is a cheat day in honor of Thor: You may have one beer, piece of chocolate or another treat.

Thor, the most famous of the Norse Gods. He is most well known as being the God of thunder and for his strength but he is also the God of the harvest and can be call upon to protect crops and to bring a bountiful harvest with his wife, Sif (who is the Goddess of the harvest). Thor is a protector of humanity and a God for the everyday working class person. He is the son of Odin and Jord, a goddess and giantess of the earth.

Now we could go into many stories of Thor and his accomplishments, but one such story, for example: Thor being challenged by Útgarða-Loki, the Giant, to drink a large drinking horn (probably full of mead) in one gulp! Thor was able to take three big gulps but was defeated, but the next day, Útgarða-Loki informed Thor that the liquid in the horn was the sea and that he would find the sea level lowered on his return trip. That would be an example of over-drinking, which is not the point of a diet! However, something can be learned from Thor's determination.

- Herbal associations - Oak, acorn, and rowen berries which are edible if cooked. They are rich in vitamin C but are sour in taste.
- What to eat? Since Thor is a bit of a glutton, you may have one cheat meal, that includes ONE beer (a full pint, 473 MLS) or your choice of a heavy carb meal.

Poem:
"God of grains/God of the farmer
Bringer of thunderstorms, benefit the
ground
Charge our garden/strength is needed for
growth
Make our crop as strong as oak
To benefit our kin"

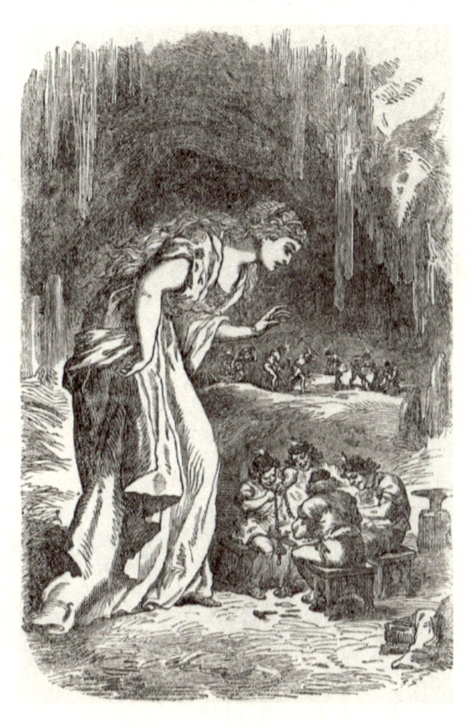

Friday

Goddesses association: Freyja and Frigg
Now there is an ongoing debate over which Goddess Friday is named after. In this book, we're not worried about that, but you may pick either Freyja or Frigg, or both? Why not!

On Friday, have one meal dedicated to your overall health and vitality that makes you feel great - listen to your body and what it's telling you, eat what it wants to eat in terms of your health. Listen to your intuition.

Freyja

- Herbal associations: Marijuana and catnip
- What to eat? Veggies and pork for one of your meals.
- What to do? Study herbs and your family tree for information on health information.

Freya or Freyja is the Goddess of magick, beauty, sexual love, war, and witchcraft. She leads the valkyries and takes half of those who die in battle to her hall, Folkvangr. She is a Vanir goddess. The Vanir are a group of ancient fertility Gods who join the Aesir after a war between the two clans.

Poem - This one focuses on breakfast.
*"Freya of the Vanir/Great of magick
Fehu to start me off
Freya of the Vanir/Teacher of magick
Empower this meal to start my day
Starting my journey of the day with (any rune at this point for your focus for the day)"*

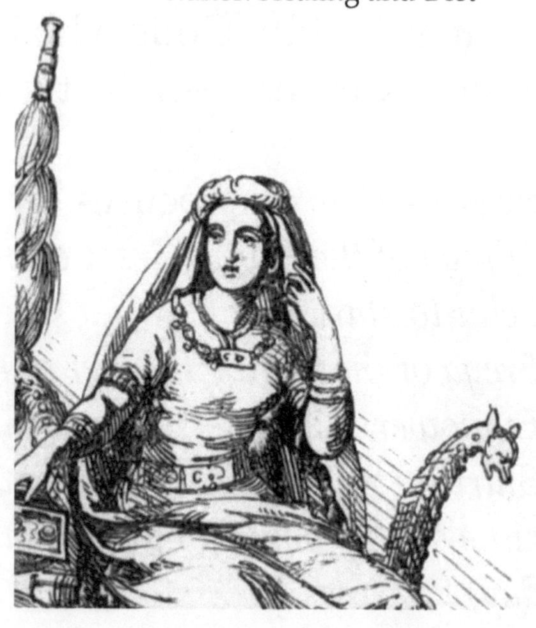

Frigg

- Herbal associations: Rose, birch, chamomile, and flax

Frigg or Frigga is the Aesir goddess of marriage, motherhood, and foresight. She is the wife of Odin and mother of Baldr.

With her gift of foresight, she was able to see the death of her son Baldr. She knew she had to stop it, so she asked everything that could be thought

to harm Baldr swear not to hurt him.
However, she didn't ask the mistletoe.
She felt the plant to be harmless, and
that fact was found out by Loki, who
then used this information to have
Hodd, the blind God, throw a mistletoe
dart at Baldr.

Poem - This one focuses on children.
"All Mother/Lady of the Aesir
Help me to provide for my children
All Mother Frigg/Wife of Odin
Who shares the throne to see all nine realms
with him.
Assist me in seeing any threats in my
children's food."

For this poem, please use Uruz in
combination with Berkana for a girl or
Teiwaz for a boy.

Saturday
God association: Hel or Hella

Now the Norse didn't have a God to pair with Saturday. The Romans named it after Saturn, who is also known as Cronos, the Titan. Some modern heathens have connected Saturday to Loki, but Freya connects Saturday with Hel or Hella.

Hel is the daughter of Loki, Goddess of the dead, ruler of her own world Helheim. Hel appears as one-half woman, the other half a skeleton. She does not let the dead leave Helheim, but she is fair and reasonable, such as in the tale of when the Gods were trying to release Baldr from Helheim. Hel said if every living thing wept for Baldr, then she would let him go, but Loki, dressed as an older woman, did not mourn, thus Baldr could not be freed from Helheim.

- Herbal associations: Potatoes or tomatoes, both are in the nightshade family.
- What to eat? Potatoes or tomatoes in one of your meals.
- What to do? Study research on GMO's and such and how to better protect your health and the health of those around you.

Hel Poem

"Hel, embracer of all
Ruler of the realm of her name
Comforter of Baldr, welcomer of all
Help me make the unknown welcoming
Perthro will be known and shared"

Daily Meal Plan Example

What does a daily meal plan look like? Here are a few examples to follow based on what I ate in a day. Please note, you can substitute vegetarian alternatives as needed, and meal times will vary for everyone. Also keep portion sizes small, but keep track of how you feel by listening to your body. If you're feeling overly hungry, increase the portion sizes.

8 am, Breakfast: Eggs with cheese (eggs cooked any way you like), and coffee with a small amount of dairy creamer.

11 am, Snack: Cheese sticks or beef jerky

2 pm, Lunch: Roasted chicken with a side of greens (my choice is green beans or cauliflower)

4 pm, Snack: Pastrami slices on water crackers

7 pm, Dinner: Pork chops with one potato or corn.

Another day, all around the same times:

Breakfast: A plate of Kerrygold cheese with coffee and a small amount of dairy creamer.

Snack: Beef jerky

Lunch: Cream cheese on bagel chips and baby carrots.

Snack: 2 hard-boiled eggs and a glass of whole milk.

Dinner: Roast beef with cauliflower (cheese on top is optional)

6. Runic Food, Vitamin and Mineral Correspondence

Fehu

It can be related to all food, vitamins, and minerals. Especially vitamin A.

Suggested rune work: Chant Fehu while brushing your hair to promote hair growth.

Uruz

Uruz is connected to vegetables and beef. It also has connections with calcium, iron, vitamin D (milk), and E (maintains muscles). Vitamin B3 - (niacin), which metabolizes energy and promotes growth, phosphorus (bones), Magnesium (bones), and Zinc (dairy).

Chant Uruz when you are sick.

Thurisaz

Since this is an aggressive rune, we can relate it to curries and chilies, pepper, and vitamin B2 (aids adrenal function)

Do not chant Thurisaz for healing purposes unless you have thoroughly studied it.

Ansuz

Ansuz food is what Freya refers to as brain food: walnut, fish, cauliflower, honey, and mushrooms. Dark chocolate as well which has flavonoids (antioxidant) which aid the brain in areas that deal with memory and learning.

Ansuz's vitamin correspondences are vitamin A for vision (prevents night blindness), B2 -vision, vitamin K (memory), vitamin E (walnuts), vitamin C (prevents mental decline and

Alzheimer's), B6 and 12 for mental health.

To work with Ansuz for health, chant it for wisdom.

Raidho

Raidho works by transporting nutrients and vitamins. Foods that are related to Raidho are any food that is quick to even out blood sugar - peanut butter or cheese are good examples of what works for me.

Vitamin E - muscles, vitamin K, Vitamin B1 (metabolism) found in pork and seeds, B6- nerve function

Chant Raidho for aid in digestion.

<u>Kenaz</u>

 Food correspondences for this rune are oranges. Also, any hot liquids such as coffee, soups, and teas. Anything that is cooked as well.

Vitamins that connect to Kenaz are vitamin C, Magnesium (regulation of temp), vitamin K as well for memory.

<u>Gebo</u>

Gebo can't be connected with any food in particular but more a meal with other people (sharing). It also relates to all vitamins.

Combine with other runes when carving on food. Such as for strength, carve Uruz and Gebo on a carrot or a piece of meat.

Wunjo

This is a rune of JOY, so a meal with other people, favorite food that is good for you, sugar in MODERATION (cane sugar) for your cheat day on Thursday. Chocolate (dark only) and licorice are also an option. A vitamin association is vitamin C and B3.

Hargalaz

Hargalaz corresponds to potatoes, eggplant, and tomatoes. Also mugwort and mushrooms,
Vitamin: potassium (found in potatoes)

Nauthiz

Nauthiz is about need. So needed vitamins and listening to what your body tells you. All vitamins and minerals due connect to this rune.

<u>Isa</u>

Isa is ice, so frozen vegetables. It can also be connected to vitamin K, which aids proper blood clotting.

<u>Jera</u>

This rune is about time. So grains and then vegetables and fruits that are in season; because this rune referrers to time! Shopping by seasonal fruits and vegetables is cost-effective too.

vitamin B1 and B2 (energy), B3 (growth), B5 (in all foods), B6- energy

<u>Eihwaz</u>

Eihwaz is the rune related to Yggdrasil, the world tree. So any fruits and also berries.

Vitamins that connect to Eihwaz are calcium, minerals, iron, vitamin D (bones), phosphorus (bones)

Perthro

Perthro is a lot cup. So it can be connected to an actual pot such as a slow cooker.

For vitamins, connect Perthro to B9 (prevents birth defects), calcium (women), folate (folic acid), vitamin D, magnesium, and iron.

Algiz

Algiz can be associated with chives, leek, onion, and garlic. Vitamins that connect to Algiz are calcium magnesium and vitamin D and C.

Chant Algiz while undergoing any kind of surgery or procedure (while you can before they put you under anesthetic)

<u>Sowulo</u>

Sowulo is the rune of the sun, so corn, sunflower seeds, chamomile, st johns wort, lemons, and oranges. Vitamins associated with this rune are vitamin D, iron, B2 (energy).

Work with Sowulos energy to boost and protect your immune system, along with Algiz and Uruz.

<u>Teiwaz</u>

Teiwaz is associated with warriors, so things that make you alert such as tea and coffee. Onions and leeks also connect to Teiwaz. Vitamins that connect to Teiwaz are iron, iodine (hormones), magnesium, and vitamin B12.

Berkana

Food associations with Berkana are broccoli and cauliflower since it looks like a tree. Also eggs (vitamin E), calcium, folic acid, and iron

Berkana can be chanted while giving birth along with Algiz, Raidho, and Sowulo for a safe and successful delivery.

Mannaz

Vitamins associated with this rune are iodine (bread), chromium, phosphorus (oats and rice and onion and garlic) vitamin K as well for memory.

Ehwaz

Ehwaz is related to animals, not just horses, so meat or tofu and beans.

Vitamins associated with Ehwaz are B12 and B9, amino acids, zinc (red meat), and iron.

Laguz

Laguz corresponds with water so that an easy connection can be made to fish, seaweed, leek, and onions. Vitamins associated with Laguz are vitamin A, Omega 3, magnesium, vitamin A (salmon), magnesium (found in blood), zinc (oysters), copper (seafood), iodine and salts (seafood), sodium from sea vegetables

Inguz

Inguz is the rune associated with the God Freyr. Freyr is the God of masculine fertility and vegetation. So foods associated with Inguz are seeds, beans sprouts, beans, eggs, honey, and nuts. Vitamins associated with this rune are vitamin E & A, magnesium and potassium, vitamin E (eggs), copper (nuts and seeds).

Othala

Othala is the rune of home, so comfort foods and also table salt!
Vitamins and minerals associated with this rune are sodium and iron (which also has protective qualities in the home, people still hang horseshoes in their homes).

Dagaz

The rune of transformation and cooking transforms food, so any food that you cook can be related to Dagaz. Vitamins related to Dagaz are C and D (Sun), and B2.

7. Diet Friendly Recipes

With this diet, each meal should have meat, fish, or animal product of some kind or another. This can be altered for those with vegetarian diets to cheese or diary and/or tofu. Then veggies, fruits (in moderation) can be added. The same moderation goes with bread, pasta or potatoes. Since this is essentially a low carb diet. You are allowed a few carbs, because it's very difficult to quit them all together, cold turkey. Sugars should also be limited. After a few weeks on this diet, I found myself having less and less craving for sugar.

<u>Cauliflower Soup</u>

Cauliflower can be associated with the brain, thus creating an easy link to Ansuz.

2 tablespoons of vegetable oil
1/2 cup of chopped onion
1 cup of chopped celery
1 whole carrot, chopped
1 medium sized cauliflower, cut into flowerets
1 tablespoon of parsley
8 cups of chicken stock
1/4 cup of butter
1/4 cup of flour
2 cups of milk
1 cup of half & half
salt to taste

<u>Bratwurst Lunch</u>

Now I could give you some complicated recipe, but for this diet, the Germans have given us the gift of bratwurst and sauerkraut. You can add red cabbage, sliced beets or okra on the side. This combo was something I grew up with in central Texas, which is an area with strong German roots.

What you'll need

1. 2 brats per person.
2. 1 onion
3. 2 beets, slided
4. 1 or 2 cups of sauerkraut, as much as you need if your serving more than one person
5. In a large pan, brown bratwurst in oil or butter and reduce heat to medium. Add onions and and cook until lightly caramelized. Remove from heat and put on a plate with sauerkraut and beets.

<u>Stampo</u>

I've decided to ad an easy to make, slow cooker friendly dish called Stampo that is Dutch in origin.

- 4 to 5 large russet or Idaho potatoes, peeled and cubed
- 4 teaspoons kosher salt
- 2 tablespoons of butter
- ½ cup 2% milk (or whole milk) or how ever much you'd like to ad for the mashed potatoes.
- 1 medium onion, chopped
- 1 or 2 carrots, chopped
- 2 large cloves garlic, peeled and minced
- 1 pound fully-cooked, smoked pork sausage such as Dutch Rookworst or Polish Kielbasa will do, cut into thin coin shaped slices

- Optional - you can ad leeks, sweet potatoes or rutabaga to your Stampo. There are multiple recipes for different types of Stampo. As long as it has potatoes, kale and sausage, it meets the requirements.

Instructions

1. Peel and chop your ingredients like the potatoes, onion and such. Then slice the leeks.

2. Place all the vegetables in a large pot, then add enough water to bring the water to a boil. Cook till tender or you can use a slow cooker for this.

3. Cook the sausage until it is browned nicely.

4. Drain the vegetables well, add butter and milk then mash

everything as you see fit. Season the dish with salt and pepper.

5. Serve with the sausage arranged on top.

Diet friendly foods to eat in a pinch-
these will leave you satisfied and keep
you on track.

- Beef jerky
- Smoked Salmon - even if your inland,
  it's easy to get and it usually is wild
  sourced. Do not eat if it is farmed
  salmon, which is practically poison.
- Cheese- cream cheese on whole wheat
  bread, cheese sticks or pre-cut cheese
  cubes.
- Salami slices, a whole pack can last me
  a week and a half at work and it's only
  $5.99
- Eggs cooked any way
- Canned Tuna

Plant based options
- Carrots
- Peanuts
- Peanut butter on toast
- Avocados

- Almonds
- Sunflower seeds
- Cucumbers
- Black and green olives
- Cauliflower
- Celery

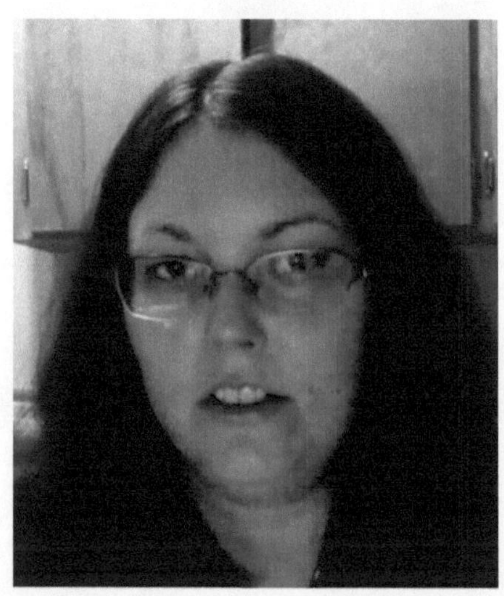

Before diet - 195 lbs taken from one of the Skype lessons I had with Freya. This was taken in September 2019

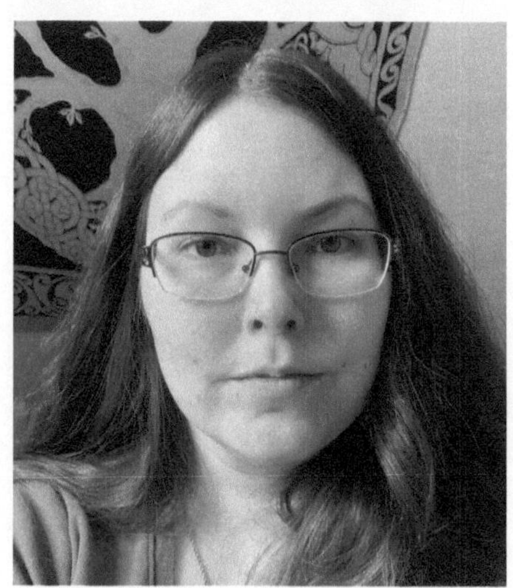

At 179 lbs, early April 2020.

8. Sigrun's Diet Diary

The second part of this book details my diet over a period of 9 weeks. This diet can be done for longer but the shortest span of time would be 9 weeks to see results. I have also included any health issues I was having and runes applicable to healing.

This diet plan is half spiritual and half physical. You will be doing both rituals/meditation and diet/exercise. The diet is not a detox diet, but focuses on calorie reduction. The calories you will eat will make you full and satisfied. Exercises will be as minimal as walking everyday or 30 minutes of heavy cardio. What is important is that you pace yourself based on your body. If you are out of shape, start slow, do not go too hard, but you must work your way up to a more intense workout in order to get results.

Keep in mind, by starting this diet, you are altering you fate, your wyrd.

Week 1: 11/17/2019- 11/23/2019.

At the start, I am 195 pounds. Quite scary since I was 235 right after I had my son Bjorn, two years ago. I had lost 55 lbs in a few months, but then put on 20 pounds.

Yuck.

Considering I am 32 years old and 5'3, and at my thinnest at 19, I was 118 pounds, this was shocking. When Freya pitched the idea of this, I was delighted. The runes have been a very motivational part of my life. I have used them for years already in magick, thanks to Freya's "Northern Mysteries and Magick." We decided on a nine-week regimen. Nine is a sacred number in the Northern tradition. Nine weeks to change my health and my body, because not only do I need to lose weight but develop a deeper understanding of the runes when used for healing.

To start my journey, I need to look at what my problems are. I'm 195 lbs, and I'm 5'3, which is very overweight for my size. I'm a busy woman; I eat a lot of processed foods, which had led me to have acne breakouts. Using my knowledge of runes, the runes I am deficient in are Jera (poor digestion) and then Dagaz, a transformation of diet.

—Later in the week—

I have had issues with back pain and arm pain. I focused on Uruz and Eihwaz, which didn't help as much as I had hoped, but I focused on Sowulo, and that helped like a hot pack. I also have had issues with my sciatic nerve in my right hip. This has been a problem for me since I was 18. I went through the Futhark in meditation for an aid. I stopped at Wunjo, because I found that it helped me tremendously.

Week 2 11/24/2019 to 11/30/2019

The runes I made my goal to focus on where Ansuz, Kenaz (light of the thought), and Mannaz this week. These runes are useful mental clarity (Freya also recommended).

I had some neck pain as well, only minor. I used Uruz to help.
For Thanksgiving, which fell on this week, I only ate with my immediate family. I ate only honey ham and pumpkin pie. My husband, Gregory, didn't want turkey this year, which made it easier.

Week 3 12/01/2019 to 12/07/2019

This week I am down to 185 lbs! But I did have some dizziness on Friday. I was visualizing Uruz to ground helped me.

Week 4: 12/08/2019-12/14/2019

This week I contracted some kind of cold: nausea and dizziness, leftover from last week. I must have picked something up from work, unfortunately. I couldn't bring myself to stand for too long. I tried Uruz and Berkana, but they did not help with the symptoms. I took a bath and visualized Laguz bringing down my fever (you don't want to use Isa for this.) I felt mentally clustered on Saturday, a bind rune of Uruz, and Algiz helped me feel a little more grounded.

Week 5 12/15/2019 to 12/21/2019

A word of advice: avoid noodles on this diet. I had made one of my favorite Italian pasta salads with smoked salmon. Just a few weeks of cutting carbs and introducing some more in made me feel horrible. Perhaps the noodles had too many processed ingredients. I recovered thanks to a car issue that required more running back and forth to check on it. I also had shoulder pain, I tried Wunjo and Uruz, but to no avail but putting my arms over my head and crossing them behind my back making a Dagaz and hold that for a few minutes really helped.

Week 6 12/22/2019- 12/28/2019

This was a good week considering it's Yule time, and there are sweets everywhere. If you've followed the diet and already lost some weight, then you've kept most of it off, and your appetite has curved as a result. The naughtiest thing I did this week was having 2 pints of Guinness, a low-calorie beer but high in carbs. Still focused on high protein and low carbs. I used Ansuz and Raidho this week to maintain focus during a sinus headache and Raidho when I was driving for a long period of time to help with blood flow to my legs.

Week 7 12/29/2019-01/04/2020

No real problems! I did quite a bit of walking this week to shed some extra pounds gained back from holiday feasts.

Week 8, 01/05/2020-01/11/2020

The biggest problem I faced this week was not with diet. No, I stubbed my pinky toe on my son's crib and broke it. I have broken my pinkie toe before, but visualizing Uruz seemed to help a bit and made it feel like I was spreading my toes, even when I wasn't .

I also had a little fever the same day, I want to say it was because of what I ate (frozen food), but I could have just gotten a small bug. I felt faint but used Uruz as well. It is important to note that I had a realization of Inguz, not to use it when treating any infection because Inguz fertilizes. Fertilization will cause bacteria growth.

Week 9, 01/12/2020-01/18/2020

I am feeling great this week! Some back problems, but meditating on Eihwaz helped.

Over these past few weeks, I've had issues with acne. Even before I started the diet, I was having acne problems like a teenager! Natural hormones could have been a culprit but now… I don't have acne! I had made an effort at the beginning of this diet to eliminate artificial sweeteners and soy. I was using soy-based nondairy creamer… what a mistake! I had switched to using milk-based creamer in my daily coffee. At the end of this week, I found myself at 180 pounds!

These next weeks were really just to continue the diary. I was already seeing results at 9 weeks which was the goal.

January 19th to 25th

I've managed to keep the weight off and curb my appetite enough to resist large meals.

January 26th to February 1st

Another fantastic week of no issues other than my sciatic nerve in my right hip acting up. Wunjo again helped to ease the discomfort.

February 2nd to 8th.

I had a dizzy spell this week, I've never experienced something like this for this long. It carried on for a good 2 minutes while I was sitting down. The room was spinning. My husband and I concluded it was the cream cheese I had for breakfast. It is quite essential to look at the food ingredients in packaged food. If there are more than 5, you're going to have problems.

February 9th to 15th

My workouts have been great; my husband has recommended a specific type for me to try. The workout consists of a lot of kicks and punches. I did manage to hurt my knee while working out, though. Uruz and Eihwaz help with the soreness and inflammation

February 16th to 22nd.

I've had to take it easy on myself with exercise this week. While I have lost weight, my body is still out of shape. Uruz and Eihwaz are always a great help when overcoming sore muscles and bones.

February 23rd to February 29th

The news has confirmed a positive case of Coronavirus in my state (Washington state). I prepared before, but extra precautions need to be taken at this time. I made additional changes to my diet to boost my immune system: Vitamin C and water and beef.

March 1st to March 7th

Continued panic over Corona Virus continues to dominate the thoughts of the people around me. In the meantime, I am preparing to move. I've spent long hours have been spent packing and getting rid of what no longer serves me. I also have quite a bit of added stress because of the house closing. I am using Raidho and Laguz to calm myself.

March 8th to 14th

My house closing has been delayed multiple times, and to top it off, my job moved us all to remote status due to fears over the Coronavirus. I am prepping not only for a move but for a lockdown. What foods are most important during a lockdown?
Water - having water jugs on hand but also have water flavor. Coffee and tea are also useful due to water fatigue.

Carbs - keep you full, not a large part of
the diet but are necessary for this
situation
Proteins - Canned animal protein is an
excellent source of vitamins.
Salt - iodized salt is essential so your
thyroid can function correctly.

It is also imperative to stay
physically active during this time. I
continue to do my workouts and to find
ways to stay entertained.

9. Further Knowledge

This section is to provide information for those more familiar with the Norse pantheon or for those who want to learn further.

11 Systems of the Body compared to the Runes

In medical science, there are now 11 recognized systems of the body, we have related the runes to all and to the 11 rivers of the Élivágar. The Élivágar rivers (translation : Ice Waves) existed in Ginnungagap and are mentioned in the Prose Edda. For a wonderful meditation, there is a powerful song by the band Heilung, where they chant the names of the 11 rivers.

1. Circulatory System - hearth, arteries and veins. Runes: Laguz, Raidho, Kenaz

Élivágar River: 'Svol - which translates to 'Ever Cold'

The circulatory system regulates temperature.

2. Digestive system: The system that is responsible for absorbing nutrients.
Runes: Jera, Fehu, Nauthiz, Dagaz
 Élivágar River: Sylgr, which translates to 'Swallower'
Waste is also associated with the digestive system, a perfect rune to associate with that is Hargalaz

3. Endocrine system: helps the body function via hormones.
Runes: Inguz, Jera, Kenaz, Teiwaz, Sowulo

Élivágar River: Vid which translates to 'wide'
Thyroid, pituitary gland, pineal gland adrenal gland, pancreas, ovary, testicles

4. Exocrine System: Skin, nails, sweat glands. Runes: Laguz

Élivágar River: Hrid, which translates to 'Snow Storm'
5. Immune and lymphatic system.
Runes: Algiz, Teiwaz, Thurisaz, Uruz
Élivágar River: Leiptr, which translates to 'Lightning'
6. Muscular system: movement
Runes: Ehwaz, Raidho, Othala, Sowulo
Élivágar River: Gunnthra- which translates to 'Battle Trough'

7. Nervous system: provides information to the senses and nerves
Runes: Ansuz, Gebo, Kenaz, Eihwaz, Ehwaz, Othala, Wunjo
Élivágar River: Ylgr, which translates to 'She wolf'
8. Renal System: includes the urinary system, the kidneys filter your blood.
Runes:
Laguz, Raido
Élivágar River: Slidr, which translates to 'Punishment'

9. Reproductive system: Inguz, Berkana, Perthro, Teiwaz
  River Fimbulthul- great roaring / another name for Odin
10. Respiratory system: a Gjoll- noisy
11. Skeletal system: Eihwaz, Algiz, Othala, Uruz
Fjorm - Hurrying

And since the feet really are not system, Freya's input is "Othala, the feet, grounded in the earth, where you live."

<u>Herbal and Food Correspondences for the Gods</u>

During the creation of this book, Freya and I came up with a whole list of herbs and foods associated with the Gods. This is for your own knowledge and benefit.

- Odin - Pine, walnuts, venison
- Freyr - Barley, honey, pork
- Njord -Sage, seaweed, fish
- Thor - Oak, acorns, pork
- Baldr - Sunflower, eye bright (also known as balers brow)
- Tyr- Yarrow, onion, leek and comfrey
- Forseti - Rosemary
- Egyr -Sea salt, fish
- Loki -Peppers
- Hemidalr- Ash, grass, buckwheat, all grains
- Hodr: Being the blind God- Mint - since it grows in little sun light

- Hermold - Since he travels to Helheim - Flax seed because help with constipation.
- Braggi - Mead and honey and barley
- Freya - Marijuana, cat nip
- Frigg - Rose, birch, chamomile and flax
- Indunn- Apple, crab apple
- Gerd - Freyr wife: Parsley, year round herb, mushrooms
- Skadi- Juniper
- Sif- Barley grass, corn, wheat, grain
- Jord - Lavender
- Nerthus- Watercress, cattail
- Gefurn, Gefjon- fennel, wheat, grain
- Gna - Apples
- Hel - Potato and tomatoes (since these are both in the nightshade family)
- Sunna - Chamomile
- Holda- Corn flower, berries

The Rune Table

This rune table was provided by a reader of the first edition, Irina Scott. This table includes Runic healing correspondences and food and vitamin correspondences for easy reference.

RUNE NAME	RUNES IN HEALING	RUNIC FOOD, VITAMIN AND MINERALS
FEHU	Digestive healing, body improvement via proper diet and exercise. Weight gain after chemo/radiation or other cases of disease-related weight loss	All food, vitamins and minerals, especially vitamin A. Chant Fehu while brushing your hair to promote hair growth.

RUNE NAME	RUNES IN HEALING	RUNIC FOOD, VITAMIN AND MINERALS
URUZ	Treating infections, even sepsis. Use to strengthen the body during and after an illness. Use it to enhance the body as you are working out. Can be used for undergoing cancer treatment.	Vegetables and beef. Calcium, iron, vitamin D (milk), E, B3, Magnesium, Zink. Chant Uruz when you sick.

RUNE NAME	RUNES IN HEALING	RUNIC FOOD, VITAMIN AND MINERALS
THURISAZ	Use for protection against an aggressive illness. Use it carefully	Curries, chilies, pepper, vitamin B2(aids adrenal function)

RUNE NAME	RUNES IN HEALING	RUNIC FOOD, VITAMIN AND MINERALS
ANSUZ	Asthma, throat issues, throat irritation, mental health	Vitamin A for vision, B2-vision, vitamin K (memory), vitamin E (walnuts), and vitamin C (prevents mental decline and Alzheimer's, B6 and B12 for mental health.

RUNE NAME	RUNES IN HEALING	RUNIC FOOD, VITAMIN AND MINERALS
RAIDHO	Blood clots (under the direct care of blood thinners). Useful for digestive issues.	Transporting nutrients and vitamins. Food that related to Raidho is food that is quick to even out blood sugar. Vitamin E- muscles, vitamin K, vitamin B1 (metabolism, found in pork & seeds)B6

RUNE NAME	RUNES IN HEALING	RUNIC FOOD, VITAMIN AND MINERALS
KENAZ	Can be used as visualization over your healthcare providers along with Ansuz.	Oranges, coffee, soups, teas. Anything that is cooked. Vitamin C, Magnesium, vitamin K (memory)

RUNE NAME	RUNES IN HEALING	RUNIC FOOD, VITAMIN AND MINERALS
GEBO	Correct diet that is nourishing the body.	Meal with other people (sharing). Related to all vitamins. Combine with other runes when carving on food. For strength carve Uruz and Gebo on a carrot or a piece of meat.

RUNE NAME	RUNES IN HEALING	RUNIC FOOD, VITAMIN AND MINERALS
WUNJO	Emotional healing and nerve pain. Works well for sciatic nerve pain.	Meal with other people, favorite food, sugar in moderation (cane sugar) for your cheat day on Thursday. Chocolate (dark only), licorice (vitamin C and B3)

RUNE NAME	RUNES IN HEALING	RUNIC FOOD, VITAMIN AND MINERALS
HAGALAZ	Point to mental diseases or diseases caused by addiction. Seek psychological healing	Potatoes, eggplant, tomatoes. Mugwort and mushrooms. Vitamin-potassium.
NAUTHIZ	Advised to assess in what needs to be done with your health.	Nauthiz is about need. Listen to your body what it needs.

RUNE NAME	RUNES IN HEALING	RUNIC FOOD, VITAMIN AND MINERALS
ISA	Halting high fever or aggressive cancers. Works on a burn.	Ice, frozen vegetables. Vitamin K, which aids proper blood clotting.

RUNE NAME	RUNES IN HEALING	RUNIC FOOD, VITAMIN AND MINERALS
JERA	Healthy gut bacteria. Healing over time (pair with appropriate rune)	This rune is about time. So grains and then vegetables and fruits that is in season. Vitamin B1, B2(energy), B3 (growth), B5 (in all foods), B6 (energy)

RUNE NAME	RUNES IN HEALING	RUNIC FOOD, VITAMIN AND MINERALS
EIHWAZ	It can be seen as a symbol of spine and within the spine the central nervous system. Can help with back and skeletal strength.	Fruits and berries. Calcium, minerals, phosphorus (bones).

RUNE NAME	RUNES IN HEALING	RUNIC FOOD, VITAMIN AND MINERALS
PERTHRO	Helpful for feminine health and a healthy menstrual cycle. Pair with Uruz, Berkana and Algiz for a safe birth.	Slow cooker. Vitamins B9 (prevents birth defects), calcium, folate (folic acid), vitamin D, magnesium, iron

RUNE NAME	RUNES IN HEALING	RUNIC FOOD, VITAMIN AND MINERALS
ALGIZ	It can protect the whole body & all its systems. Offers protection against disease & medical malpractice. Pair with appropriate rune (for example when going in for surgery).	Chives, leek, onion, garlic. Vitamins-calcium magnesium, vitamin D and C. Chant Algiz while undergoing any kind of surgery or procedure (while you can before they put you under anesthetic).

RUNE NAME	RUNES IN HEALING	RUNIC FOOD, VITAMIN AND MINERALS
SOWULO	Health in general, life force and Vitamin D3).	Corn, sunflower seeds, chamomile, St. John's wort, lemons, oranges. Vitamins D, iron, B2. Use to boost & protect your immune system, along with Algiz and Uruz.

RUNE NAME	RUNES IN HEALING	RUNIC FOOD, VITAMIN AND MINERALS
TEIWAZ	Fighting cancer and therapy that involves male fertility issues and injectable medications ones immune system.	Tea, coffee, onions, leeks. Vitamins – iron, iodine (hormones), magnesium, vitamin B12.

RUNE NAME	RUNES IN HEALING	RUNIC FOOD, VITAMIN AND MINERALS
BERKANA	Female fertility and breast health	Broccoli, cauliflower, eggs (vitamin E), calcium, folic acid, iron. Berkana can be chanted while giving birth along with Algiz, Raidho, Sowulo for a safe and successful delivery.

RUNE NAME	RUNES IN HEALING	RUNIC FOOD, VITAMIN AND MINERALS
EHWAZ	Healthy movement of bowels and muscles.	Meat, tofu, beans. Vitamins B12, B9, amino acids, zinc (red meat), iron.

RUNE NAME	RUNES IN HEALING	RUNIC FOOD, VITAMIN AND MINERALS
MANNAZ	Mental relationship changes or treatment. Parkinson's disease, treating nerve damage (pair with Ansuz or Ehwaz).	Iodine (bread), chromium, phosphorus (oats, rice, onions, garlic). Vitamin K (for memory).

RUNE NAME	RUNES IN HEALING	RUNIC FOOD, VITAMIN AND MINERALS
LAGUZ	Emotional issues and resolving blood clots in addition to medication.	Fish, seaweed, leek, onions. Vitamins A, omega3, magnesium (found in blood), zinc (oysters), copper (seafood), sodium from sea vegetables

RUNE NAME	RUNES IN HEALING	RUNIC FOOD, VITAMIN AND MINERALS
INGUZ	Potent male fertility, fertility treatment for males and prostate health.	God Freyr. Masculine fertility and vegetation. Seeds, beans, sprouts, beans, eggs, honey, nuts. Vitamin E, A, magnesium, potassium, vitamin E (eggs), copper (nuts and seeds).

RUNE NAME	RUNES IN HEALING	RUNIC FOOD, VITAMIN AND MINERALS
OTHALA	Family disease, such as cancers that run in the family. Also, positive family health attributes.	Vitamins and minerals are sodium, iron (which also has protective qualities in the home).

RUNE NAME	RUNES IN HEALING	RUNIC FOOD, VITAMIN AND MINERALS
DAGAZ	Psychical transformation from a healthy diet. Useful for diet change, lifestyle change.	Any food that you cook. Vitamins C, D (sun), B12.

Further Reading

For those interested in more in depth knowledge on the runes and the Norse pantheon, please check out these books:

"Northern Mysteries and Magick" by Freya Aswynn

"Leaves of Yggdrasil" by Freya Aswynn

"Futhark A Handbook of Rune Magic" by Edred Thorsson

"Runelore" by Edred Thorsson

"Prose Edda" by Snorri Sturlson

"The Poetic Edda" - author unknown but there are translations available for free online.

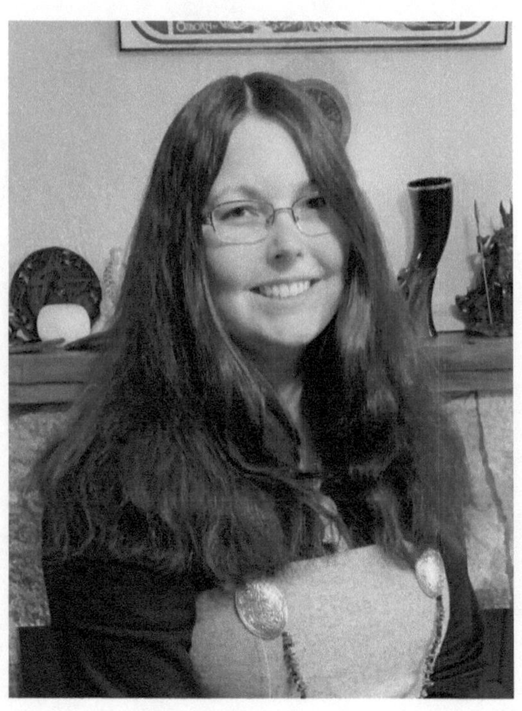

About the author:

Sigrún Gregerson is a student of Freya Aswynn. She has been studying the runes under Freya and on her own since 2016. Her knowledge of runes not only includes health and healing, but general magick as well. She currently lives in Washington state with her husband and son.